100 Questions & Answers About Migraine

Second Edition

Katherine A. Henry, MD

Associate Professor of Neurology
New York University School of Medicine
Chief of Neurology
Bellevue Hospital Center
New York, NY

Anthony P. Bossis, PhD

Clinical Assistant Professor of Psychiatry and Anesthesiology
New York University School of Medicine
Co-Director, Pain Management Center
Bellevue Hospital Center
New York, NY

JONES AND BARTLETT PUBLISHERS
Sudbury, Massachusetts
BOSTON   TORONTO   LONDON   SINGAPORE

World Headquarters
Jones and Bartlett Publishers
40 Tall Pine Drive
Sudbury, MA 01776
978-443-5000
info@jbpub.com
www.jbpub.com

Jones and Bartlett Publishers
Canada
6339 Ormindale Way
Mississauga, Ontario L5V 1J2
Canada

Jones and Bartlett Publishers
International
Barb House, Barb Mews
London W6 7PA
United Kingdom

Jones and Bartlett's books and products are available through most bookstores and online booksellers. To contact Jones and Bartlett Publishers directly, call 800-832-0034, fax 978-443-8000, or visit our website, www.jbpub.com.

Substantial discounts on bulk quantities of Jones and Bartlett's publications are available to corporations, professional associations, and other qualified organizations. For details and specific discount information, contact the special sales department at Jones and Bartlett via the above contact information or send an email to specialsales@jbpub.com.

The authors, editor, and publisher have made every effort to provide accurate information. However, they are not responsible for errors, omissions, or for any outcomes related to the use of the contents of this book and take no responsibility for the use of the products and procedures described. Treatments and side effects described in this book may not be applicable to all people; likewise, some people may require a dose or experience a side effect that is not described herein. Drugs and medical devices are discussed that may have limited availability controlled by the Food and Drug Administration (FDA) for use only in a research study or clinical trial. Research, clinical practice, and government regulations often change the accepted standard in this field. When consideration is being given to use of any drug in the clinical setting, the healthcare provider or reader is responsible for determining FDA status of the drug, reading the package insert, and reviewing prescribing information for the most up-to-date recommendations on dose, precautions, and contraindications, and determining the appropriate usage for the product. This is especially important in the case of drugs that are new or seldom used.

Production Credits

Senior Acquisitions Editor: Nancy Anastasi Duffy
Senior Editorial Assistant: Jessica Acox
Production Director: Amy Rose
Production Assistant: Laura Almozara
Marketing Manager: Ilana Goddess

V.P. of Manufacturing and Inventory Control:
 Therese Connell
Composition: Spoke & Wheel/Jason Miranda
Printing and Binding: Malloy, Inc.

Cover Credits

Cover Design: Kristin E. Ohlin, Carolyn Downer
Cover Image: Top left: © @erics/ShutterStock, Inc.; Top right: © Victoria Alexandrova/ShutterStock, Inc.;
 Bottom left: © Rene Jansa/ShutterStock, Inc.; Bottom right: © Gary Paul Lewis/ShutterStock, Inc.
Cover Printing: Malloy, Inc.

Library of Congress Cataloging-in-Publication Data

Henry, Katherine A.
 100 questions & answers about migraine / Katherine A. Henry, Anthony P. Bossis.—2nd ed.
  p. cm.
 Includes bibliographical references and index.
 ISBN-13: 978-0-7637-6412-8 (alk. paper)
 ISBN-10: 0-7637-6412-4 (alk. paper)
 1. Migraine—Popular works. 2. Migraine—Miscellanea. I. Bossis, Anthony P. II. Title. III. Title: 100 questions and answers about migraine. IV. Title: One hundred questions and answers about migraine.

 RC392.H45 2009
 616.8'4912—dc22

                    2008036080

6048

Printed in the United States of America
13 12 11 10 09   10 9 8 7 6 5 4 3 2

CONTENTS

In the three years since our first edition, we have been gratified by the knowledge and comfort that our book has brought to our patients, friends, coworkers, and family members. We are pleased that we are reaching those individuals who suffer—often unbearably—from headaches in their everyday lives.

Migraine affects 13% of adults in the United States. Nearly 1 in 5 women and 1 in 20 men suffer from this disabling disease, making migraine one of the major health issues of our time. Further, migraine affects individuals during the prime of their lives, when they are most intensely involved with their families and careers. The time we have to spend with our patients is small in comparison to the amount of time they spend coping with the illness.

It is our hope that our book will continue to bridge this gap. Knowledge is empowering when it comes to your medical problems. It also helps to know you are not alone. In this text, we have created a series of questions and answers that will allow you to better understand your migraines and put you back in control of your life.

Many of the questions and answers have been updated to include recent research findings to migraine and their relevance to your care. Several of the questions have been reordered and expanded to improve their flow and breadth.

In preparing the second edition, once again we would like to first and foremost thank our patients. Without them we could not have written this book. Their questions and concerns guided us in putting together a book that is relevant to their concerns. Specifically, our migraineurs, Cherie Spitzer and Max Veron, offered superb comments that illustrate the experiences of many persons with migraines. Thanks also go to our many readers who have given us their feedback and comments on the first edition. Finally, we would like to thank our families, Carl and Zack, and Lauren and Julia, whose patience and support have been invaluable.

Katherine Henry, MD
Anthony Bossis, PhD

The best little compact resource for headache sufferers just got better. While the most important questions have (and should) remain the same, in their *Second Edition* of *100 Questions & Answers About Migraine*, Henry and Bossis have expanded, updated, and "perfected" their answers based on a combination of reflection and advances in knowledge based on research. Since the first edition was released, patients to whom I have referred the book have found it invaluable. The breadth and scope of material serves as learning resource, a springboard for communicating with their physicians during follow-up visits, and a guide to self-efficacy—managing their illness and improving their health-related quality of life. I have also referred my student physicians to this book since headache is the most common neurological complaint in the clinical practice of neurologists, and patients will be asking them these very questions for the rest of their career.

There have been plenty of books on headache and migraine written for patients by very knowledgeable and experienced physicians and other healthcare professionals that are well researched and replete with important information. However, the singular feature that makes this volume unique is the *accessible* format of questions and answers. Readers do not have to sift through a complete volume to find the pearls or answers to the questions that are most important and relevant to them.

This book is not just about headache. The authors' deft and balanced approach to the integration of exercise, complementary and alternative medicine, and stress-reducing techniques (along with photographs of actual migraine prevention exercises) provides patients with abundant tips to enhance wellness and ameliorate other chronic medical disorders.

My congratulations to Drs. Henry and Bossis on their second edition and what I hope to be a continually updated volume as knowledge and therapeutics advance.

David W. Dodick, MD
Professor, Department of Neurology
Mayo Clinic

As a physician who had worked with migraine patients for many years, I would like to begin by complimenting the authors on a unique, well written, comprehensive, and valuable resource for migraine sufferers and their families. What I particularly like about *100 Questions & Answers About Migraine* is the question-and-answer style and the skill with which the authors handle many of the challenging questions that patients ask. Drs. Henry and Bossis truly empower patients with this book by giving them the information, resources, references, and all the options that are available to them to take control of their chronic illness.

Another point emphasized in the book is the need for physicians and patients to move away from thinking of migraine as a "pain syndrome" rather than a complex neurological disorder with multiple clinical manifestations, which alone or collectively may be as disabling as the pain itself. This paradigm shift in our concept of this illness, together with a valuable and insightful section on coping with migraine, makes this a particularly useful resource for those migraineurs who struggle with the emotional and physical aspects of this often-disabling disease.

I especially like their approach to the emotional side of migraine and complementary and alternative medicines (Parts 5 and 6). I believe that most physicians and patients will benefit from their balanced approach and find the description of "wellness" and the interaction between stress, depression, anxiety, and headaches important and useful. Their discussion of complementary and alternative medicine is especially timely given the increasing interest that many patients have in these approaches to managing chronic illness. It is unusual to find a patient education book that so adeptly addresses the issues that are important to our patients.

Again, my congratulations to Drs. Henry and Bossis on an extremely well written book and what I am sure will be an outstanding resource and self-help guide for patients, their families, and their physicians.

David W. Dodick, MD
Mayo Clinic, Scottsdale, Arizona

PART ONE

All About Migraine

What is the history of migraine?

What is a migraine?

What are the changes that occur in the brain
that lead to migraine?

What causes migraine?

More . . .

1. What is the history of migraine?

Many famous historical figures have suffered from migraine. Notable migraineurs include Julius Caesar, Vincent van Gogh, Napoleon, Lewis Carroll, President Thomas Jefferson, Sigmund Freud, Virginia Woolf, and Elvis Presley, to name a few. The first descriptions of headache are thought to date back to 3000 B.C., and through the centuries the descriptions of migraine have been remarkably similar, with historical writings referring to the severe pain, nausea, visual symptoms, and physical prostration brought on by a migraine. Hippocrates, often called the "father of medicine," was one of the first to describe the visual auras accompanying headache as early as 300 B.C., and he was probably the first to describe the role of triggers in precipitating migraine attacks.

Hemicrania

Half of the brain or head. May also refer to one of the cerebral hemispheres.

The term *migraine* stems from the word **hemicrania**, meaning half of the head or brain, and was first used in the second century A.D. by Galenus of Pergamon. Early theories postulated that migraine originated from circulating "humors or vapours," and it was not until the 1700s that the concept of vasodilation (widening of the blood vessels) of the blood vessels surrounding the brain was put forth. Only in the last decade or so have we recognized the importance of certain brain structures and neurotransmitters (chemical messengers in the nervous system) as players in the cascade of events leading to a migraine. The advances in genetics and neurobiology have allowed us to very rapidly make new discoveries about the pathogenesis of migraines and their treatment.

2. What is a migraine?

Chances are if you picked up this book, you are one of the millions of Americans who suffer from migraine headaches. Migraine is one of the most severe types of headache pain and one of the most severe types of pain in the human experience. Many who have migraine are not aware this is the disease causing their suffering. If you already know that you have migraine, you may worry about brain tumors and life-threatening neurological problems when the pain of a migraine grabs you. It is not uncommon to feel helpless and frustrated when the pain of a migraine seems to go on and on, and to wonder if migraine is really the correct diagnosis.

It is not uncommon to feel helpless and frustrated when the pain of a migraine seems to go on and on.

Migraine is a neurological illness that is the not-so-nice end result of the dovetailing of genetics, emotions, neurobiology, and the environment. This type of headache is unlike the typical mild headache most people have every now and again. Migraine headaches may cause you to take to your bed, turn off the lights, lie still, and ban all noise and activity from your vicinity. You may not be able to work, or take care of your house or children, and you may find that you are so ill that you vomit or wish that you could. You may also experience diarrhea and fatigue and an inability to concentrate. All of this is in addition to the severe throbbing pain that may take over one side or most of your head. If you are a migraine sufferer, you may have only the occasional attack or you may have headaches several times a month. You may find a close association with your menstrual periods if you are a woman, or certain foods or environmental factors such as odors or the weather, or you may feel as though the headaches come on with no particular pattern.

Migraines are often so painful that you may feel as though what you are experiencing cannot "just be a headache." You may feel this way when you are experiencing a bout of particularly troublesome or persistent migraines, even though you have had them for years.

3. What are the changes that occur in the brain that lead to migraine?

You may find it frustrating to have severe migraines and yet be told over and over that everything appears "normal." Migraine sufferers are often left feeling misunderstood and maligned as they spend hours or days in bed unable to function from a disorder that has no visible medical manifestation to the outside world. When we see patients in the clinic, we expect them to have a normal neurological examination and essentially normal brain imaging. However, we are well aware that fundamental neurochemical processes are taking place that lead to severe pain for the migraineur.

Migraine is a scientific arena where great advances have been made over the last decade. This has led to the development of an enhanced understanding of the disorder and much more specific and effective medications. Neurobiology is one of the most fascinating areas of human anatomy and physiology. The pathophysiology of migraine calls into play the various levels of complexity of the nervous system.

Vasodilation

Expansion of blood vessels.

Historically, it was believed that the pain of migraine resulted from an expansion of the large blood vessels (called **vasodilation**) supplying the brain. This expansion led to a stretching of the nerve fibers attached to these vessels, which led to the perception of pain. Treatments were aimed at constricting these blood vessels.

In the early 1990s, experiments were performed showing that when these nerves are activated, they also release neurotransmitters that cause dilation and inflammation of blood vessels. This interaction between neurotransmitters and the blood vessels is felt to take place in the

trigemino-vascular junction. The nerve fibers that surround the blood vessels are branches of the trigeminal nerve. When they are activated, electrical impulses travel along the trigeminal nerve into the lower **brain stem**, which is the most primitive portion of the brain (**Figure 1**). The brain stem is about the size of your thumb, but many important functions take place in this area of the **central nervous system** (CNS). The trigeminal nerve has three branches: the ophthalmic division, which supplies the area around the eye and the forehead; the maxillary division, which supplies the cheek and the upper jaw; and the mandibular division, which supplies the lower jaw. This information is then passed on to cells that also receive information from the head, face, scalp, sinuses, and neck.

Trigemino-vascular junction

The system in the brain and brain stem that has been discovered to be the heart of the migraine generator. Neurochemical processes are believed to begin here and lead to the neurochemical cascade resulting in a migraine.

Brain stem

A portion of the brain that is relatively primitive and controls the nerves that control facial expression, swallowing, hearing, eye movements, and sensation of the face and mouth. This part of the brain is believed to be implicated in the genesis of migraines.

Central nervous system

The portion of the nervous system located in the spinal column and skull. It includes the brain and cranial nerves and spinal cord.

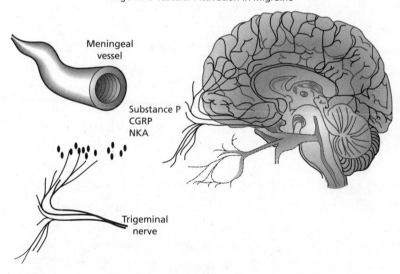

Trigemino-vascular Activation in Migraine

Meningeal vessel

Substance P
CGRP
NKA

Trigeminal nerve

Figure 1 Diagram of the brain showing the cortex, blood vessels, brain stem, trigemino-vascular system, and other structures associated with migraines.

Once the cascade is started, it is easy to see how many of the symptoms that plague migraine sufferers come about. Many migraineurs have neck pain, scalp tenderness, facial pain, eye swelling, tearing, and nasal dripping. Many of these symptoms are frightening to sufferers but are actually logical if you understand the anatomy of the migraine and how the pain blossoms and travels.

Neurons

The cells in the nervous system.

Currently scientists believe that the **neurons** in the brain are hyper-excitable in between migraine attacks, and that this hyper-excitable state makes these cells more susceptible to the processes leading to a migraine. The membranes surrounding these cells have microscopic channels through which electrolytes pass and to which neurotransmitters attach, leading to a series of chemical reactions. When these channels are abnormal, it is referred to as a **channelopathy**. It has been suggested that migraine may be a type of channelopathy. These channelopathies make the neurons unstable and susceptible to spontaneous activation or dysfunction. If this dysfunction occurs on the surface of the brain, a slowly moving electrical "wave" may spread across the brain. This phenomenon, which is referred to as **spreading cortical depression**, is experienced as an aura by many people. An aura may be accompanied by flashing or jagged lights moving slowly across the field of vision. Cortical spreading depression is capable of activating trigeminal nerve fibers, a mechanism that explains why headache often occurs after the aura has started. It is not known at this time how the trigeminal system is activated in the absence of an aura, but researchers are busy trying to answer this question.

Channelopathy

An abnormality in the membranes of neurons, the cells in the brain, making them more excitable and susceptible to migraine triggers.

Spreading cortical depression

A phenomenon seen in brain cells in which their activity becomes depressed immediately prior to the onset of the pain of a headache.

Calcitonin gene-related peptide

A neuropeptide that acts as a neuro-transmitter to dilate blood vessels.

Many substances and receptors play roles in the propagation of a migraine. **Calcitonin gene-related peptide**

(CGRP) is known to be released from trigeminal nerve endings during a migraine attack. This neurotransmitter is thought to be the main culprit in causing the dilation of blood vessels. Among the most important receptors are the **serotonin or 5-hydroxytryptamine (5-HT) receptors** that sit on the blood vessels and tips of the trigeminal nerve endings. Newer drugs used to treat migraine, the so-called **triptans**, specifically attach to these 5-HT receptors, leading to the constriction of blood vessels.

Serotonin or 5-hydroxytryp-tamine (5-HT) receptor

The receptor for serotonin. It is very important in the migraine neurochemical pain cascade.

Triptans

A revolutionary class of medications that act at the serotonin receptors to alleviate migraine pain.

For many years, headaches were believed to be a psychological manifestation of neuroticism or to reflect a character weakness in the individual. The scientific and genetic advances in understanding migraine have led us away from blaming the victim and yielded treatments that have revolutionized the management of this devastating pain syndrome. Not surprisingly, once migraine gained scientific credibility as a neurological disease, more attention and resources were aimed at better understanding the science and management of this disabling disorder.

4. What causes migraine?

Historically, headaches were believed to happen only occasionally, so they were often referred to as a paroxysmal disorder—that is, an intermittently occurring condition. Now that more is known about the genetics of migraine, this belief has been somewhat modified. Currently, neurologists believe that migraine is actually a chronic disease with intermittent headaches that vary in their degree of pain and disability. While it is unknown what specifically causes a migraine in a particular person, it is generally thought that many factors come together to trigger a migraine attack. These

Triggers

Specific events or conditions that may provoke a migraine episode. They may include certain foods, stress, weather conditions, and travel, among many other possibilities.

factors, called **triggers**, may be stress or food related, hormonal, or environmental, to name a few. These triggers activate the neurochemical cascade described in Question 3, leading to a migraine. So, if your genetic make-up puts you more at risk for migraine, exposure to multiple triggers might lead to a headache.

Initially it may be difficult, if not impossible, to identify triggers. You should try your best to scan your environment and lifestyle for possible triggers. Some of us have difficulty admitting that we are stressed out, do not get enough sleep, drink alcohol, and/or eat certain foods even when we know they cause headaches. Nevertheless, all is not lost if your search for triggers is not fruitful. While prevention or avoiding triggers is the best way to decrease your migraine attacks, treatments are available to relieve pain when migraine strikes. Questions 54 to 57 address triggers in much greater detail.

5. I think I have migraines, but sometimes I wonder if something else is causing my headaches. What are some of the other causes of headache?

Many medical problems may cause headache, such as poorly controlled high blood pressure or diabetes, anemia, human immunodeficiency virus (HIV), infection, and chronic renal failure. If you have any of these medical problems and are suffering from headaches, you may wish to discuss the issue with your physician and consider consultation with a neurologist. Headaches in conjunction with various medical problems may be the result of your body adjusting to your underlying disease or may be a reaction to the various medications used to treat your medical problems.

You may also experience headaches after cardiac bypass surgery or other types of heart or lung surgery where you are placed on a bypass machine. The cause of these headaches is not known, but they are usually treated with the same medications used for tension headaches.

Pain in the **temporo-mandibular joint** (where the jaw meets the skull) is also known to trigger more generalized tension or migraine headache and is the result of a misalignment of the jaw bone into the skull. Pain is usually felt in the teeth and jaw and may radiate outward, resulting in diffuse pain and headache. **Bruxism** (grinding of the teeth) is also associated with this condition. Grinding of the teeth or other misalignment of the jaw and temporo-mandibular joint may stimulate the branches of the trigeminal nerve and precipitate a migraine. If this disorder is suspected, you may be referred to a dentist or a physician specializing in temporo-mandibular problems. These specialists may recommend a mouth guard or dental device to relieve night-time clenching of the jaw and bruxism.

Temporo-mandibular joint
The joint where the jaw meets the skull.

Bruxism
Grinding or clenching of the teeth, usually at night.

Another condition often confused with migraine is sinus headache. Often, headaches that are thought to be a result of sinus infection are, in fact, migrainous. They may actually be related because the structures involved in migraine are located directly behind the sinuses. Inflamed sinuses may precipitate a migraine; conversely, migraine is known to occur with fullness of the sinuses and a runny nose. However, one is usually predominant. Both conditions are very common, so you should rely on your physician to make the distinction. Your primary care physician can differentiate between migraine and sinus headaches after a careful history and physical examination. Sinus headaches are usually accompanied by a purulent (greenish or yellowish)

Frontal and maxillary sinuses

Spaces in the bones of the face above the eyes (frontal) and below the eyes (maxillary) that may become congested and lead to infection and subsequent sinus headaches. These headaches are often confused with migraine headaches.

discharge or mucus. A fever is usually present, as well as pressure or pain over the **frontal and maxillary sinuses** (**Figure 2**). It is important that sinus headaches are not overdiagnosed and treated with antibiotics. Given the frequency of headaches in the general population and the rapidity with which we become resistant to antibiotics, it is important that we not take antibiotics that we do not need. Misdiagnosing a migraine as a sinus headache will lead to a delay in the appropriate treatment of migraine as well as unnecessary diagnostic and/or surgical procedures.

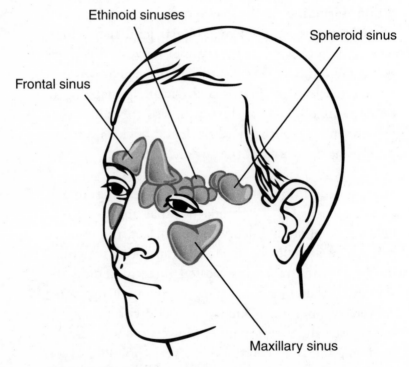

Ethinoid sinuses

Spheroid sinus

Frontal sinus

Maxillary sinus

Figure 2 The sinuses.

6. *What are some of the neurological diseases that cause secondary headaches?*

Several neurological disorders are accompanied by headaches.

- **Post-concussive headaches:** Head trauma is very common in our society. If you have had any head injury with loss of consciousness or a loss of memory for the event (concussion), you may notice a myriad of symptoms for weeks to months after the initial event. Headache is one of the most common symptoms in such cases. These headaches may be initially troubling but gradually fade with mild analgesics in most people. It is very important that you are evaluated by a physician following head trauma to rule out dangerous blood clots in the brain. This is especially true if you lose consciousness. Even if you initially feel well and develop a headache, you should see a physician for evaluation, as blood clots may develop slowly. If you are already predisposed to migraines because of family history, you may find that you begin to have migraines following minor head trauma.

- **Tumors:** The issue of tumors and headaches is discussed at length in Question 16. While it is unlikely that you are harboring a dangerous tumor, the fear of tumors is certainly stressful. You should discuss your concerns with your physician and make sure that your questions are answered to your satisfaction.

- **Cervicogenic headaches:** These headaches arise from the neck and usually result from arthritis, trauma to the neck, and muscle spasm. All of these conditions may lead to changes in the mechanics of the neck bones and musculature, resulting in headache. Migraines themselves also may lead to

Cervicogenic
Headaches that emanate from the irritation of nerves in the neck.

11

tension through the shoulder and neck muscles, resulting in a vicious cycle of spasm and headache that is very difficult to break. (See "Feature: Exercises for Migraine Prevention" on page 223.)

(See "Feature: Exercises for Migraine Prevention" on page 223.)

Arteriovenous malformation (AVM)

An abnormal tangle of blood vessels, arteries and veins in the brain. AVMs may bleed, cause seizures, focal neurological deficits, migraines, or no symptoms at all.

- **Arteriovenous malformation:** Blood vessels in the brain may be abnormal from birth, and over time these vessels become engorged and less efficient in their function. These malformations may lead to headaches and in some cases rupture, leading to minor or even catastrophic bleeding in the brain. This is one of the disorders that neurologists are ruling out when they order magnetic resonance imaging (MRI) or a computerized axial tomography (CAT or CT) scan of your brain. Many people live normal lives with these malformations and never know they have them. These days, many options are available for treating these lesions if their location is accessible. For example, physicians may embolize (or clog) the vessels, surgically remove them, or apply radiation to the area.

- **Cerebral aneurysm:** A cerebral aneurysm is a small out-pouching of a vessel in the brain. While aneurysms are not uncommon, they do not rupture at a very high rate. When they do rupture and bleed, they produce sudden, severe headache and often are accompanied by loss of consciousness. These symptoms are considered "danger signals" and should be taken very seriously. If treated quickly, outcomes are much better than if you wait. These aneurysms are usually "clipped" around the neck of the out-pouching, thereby closing off the weak portion of the vessel. Although many of us have aneurysms in our heads, they leak or burst only very rarely. When people worry about having something seriously wrong causing their headache, they tend to worry first about tumors and then about cerebral aneurysms.

- **Epilepsy:** Seizures are often followed by headaches, but it is unusual for a person with epilepsy to have headache as a presenting symptom of the epilepsy. When a person has epilepsy, headaches usually come on in the minutes following a seizure and dissipate either on their own or with mild analgesics.

- **Postoperatively, following brain surgery:** Some patients report headaches following brain surgery, regardless of whether headaches were present before the surgery. Often patients will complain of pain, tingling, or burning around the surgical scar. Sometimes if the person has risk factors for migraine, the headaches may be migrainous, but usually they are nonspecific. These headaches can be treated with the medicines used for tension headache or migraine headache.

- **Post-infectious headaches:** You may experience headaches following **viral meningitis** or encephalitis. Meningitis is an infection of the **meninges**, the tissues surrounding the brain. **Encephalitis** is an infection of the brain itself. Following treatment of the infection, some people have persistent headaches. These headaches are often treated with mild analgesics with good success.

- **Pseudotumor cerebri:** Also called **benign intracranial hypertension**, this headache is the result of increased pressure in the brain, but the cause is unknown. While there are many possible causes of this disorder, often no specific etiology is discovered. This disease predominantly affects overweight young women, and its hallmark is a change in the nerve in the back of the eye and a headache not typical of tension or migraine headache.

Viral meningitis

A viral infection of the tissues surrounding the brain.

Meninges

The tissues that envelope the brain matter. These tissues protect the brain, but may also become infected with viruses and bacteria leading to meningitis.

Encephalitis

An infection of the brain matter.

Benign intracranial hypertension

A headache disorder characterized by increased pressure in the brain, often treated by removing cerebrospinal fluid. This disorder is usually accompanied by blurring of vision. Individuals with this condition are often overweight and female.

13

Treatment usually consists of pain control, weight loss, and certain medications to lower the pressure on the brain. If vision is threatened, eye surgery may be necessary. Spinal taps may also be used to relieve pressure.

This list is by no means exhaustive. If you have been diagnosed with a neurological disorder and are wondering whether headaches are a side effect of this disorder, speak with your physician or log on to the American Academy of Neurology website at *http://www.aan.com* for more patient information or the American Headache Society, *http://www.ahsnet.org* or *http://www.achenet.org*.

7. *Who gets migraines?*

An estimated 28 million Americans suffer from migraine. Measuring the **prevalence** of a disease in a population is a difficult task. Usually researchers interview very large numbers of individuals and determine how many have migraine. The people interviewed number in the tens of thousands, and the data collected in this way allow researchers to estimate the proportion of people in a given population who have a disease—in this case migraine—during a specified period of time. This proportion is the prevalence, expressed as a ratio (1 in 1000, 1 in 150,000, and so on). Many studies have been done in the United States and throughout the world on the prevalence of migraine. However, the prevalence varies by race and geography, and it is believed that these differences support the theory that migraine is a genetically determined disease.

Asian Americans have the lowest prevalence of migraine, followed by African Americans. The highest prevalence of migraine is seen in Caucasians, including Hispanics.

Prevalence

The number of people who have a disease at any given point in time as a proportion of the total population.

In the United States, migraine is a very common disorder and is seen in 18% to 20% of women compared to 6% to 8% of men, or 13% of all adults. In other words, approximately one in five women suffers from migraine. Whether you are a man or a woman, clearly you are not alone in your struggle with severe headaches. Migraine is a common disorder.

Age also influences the prevalence of migraine for women. The prevalence of migraine in women tends to increase from puberty to age 45 or so, but then decreases gradually after menopause. Men tend to have a minimal increase in prevalence during the same time period, with a decrease in later life.

As income or education level increases, the prevalence of migraine decreases. This is in contradiction to the previously held belief that migraine was more common in higher-income groups. It is now thought that because higher-income individuals have more access to health care, they were disproportionately represented in earlier studies that mainly counted the number of patients with a given diagnosis who made doctor visits. Modern methodologies for determining prevalence ensure adequate sampling of a cross section of people of all ages, races, educational levels, and income levels. These broader data have enabled us to paint a more accurate picture of who suffers from migraine in the United States. The revised concept of prevalence does not mean that people with high education levels or incomes do not get migraines; rather, it simply means that proportionately they are not the majority.

Migraine accounts for expenditures of more than $12 billion for treatment (direct costs) and more than $13 billion annually due to lost days of work and decreased productivity (indirect costs). The latter figure is probably not a surprise to you if you have missed days of work because of your headaches or if you have been less than productive while on the job and suffering from a migraine.

Have you ever wondered if your physician can truly relate to your pain or your medical problem? Well, in the case of migraine, it is very probable that your neurologist is perfectly able to do so. A recent study of neurologists participating in a headache review course revealed that the lifetime prevalence of migraine in male neurologists was more than 30%; in male neurologists specializing in headache, it was more than 40%. In female neurologists, the lifetime prevalence was more than 60%; for female headache specialists, it was more than 80%. Migraine is one of the few medical diseases where you have a very strong likelihood of being taken care of by a physician who knows exactly what you are going through and has probably taken many of the medications, experienced the side effects, lived through the intense pain, and can truly **empathize** with you and your predicament. It is unlikely that your neurologist will share this information with you because the focus of your visit is on *your* migraine, but it does mean that you may very well be partnering in your treatment with a fellow sufferer.

Empathize

The ability to relate to what another person feels or is going through.

8. Are migraines inherited? What is the likelihood that my children will have them?

Cherie's comment:

As a child I suffered from headaches, and I can remember being in school and wishing I could be home in my comfy bed with my familiar blanket wrapped around me. I guess that was my own soothing mechanism at the time, which I used as a form of visualization. My headaches were not diagnosed as "migraines" until I was in my forties.

It is clear that migraine runs in families. While physicians know this fact intuitively from our practices caring for people with migraine, little research has actually been done in this area. Some of the largest population studies have come from the Netherlands, where it was found that first-degree relatives of migraineurs with aura were 3.8 times more likely to have migraine than the general population. **Monozygotic** (identical) **twin** studies have not been 100% conclusive but do show that it is highly likely that if one twin has migraine, the other twin will as well. A rare form of migraine with aura, **familial hemiplegic migraine**, has actually been linked to a specific chromosome. While this form of migraine occurs in very few individuals, it has provided researchers with a wealth of information about the genetics of migraine.

It is difficult to predict exactly whether your children will be affected. One point of view is that the potential for migraine is present in everyone but that genetics and environmental triggers play a role in setting off a volley of events leading to the migraine and its sequelae (aftereffects). Therefore, if you are a migraineur, your children have a higher risk than the general population. While this burden may seem onerous, keep in mind that if you have mastered the lifestyle changes that keep your migraines at bay, then your children will be raised in an environment where triggers are minimized. Migraines also will not be an unusual nor alarming event for your children if you have learned to live with them; therefore, migraines' impact may be lessened on your children as you help them adjust.

Until we understand more about the various channelopathies described in Question 3 and other familial disorders whose genetic make-up results in the disorder we know as migraine, we will not be able to accurately

It is clear that migraine runs in families.

Monozygotic twin

Twins who share the same sex and genetic constitution; identical twins.

Familial hemiplegic migraine

A rare inherited form of migraine characterized by weakness on one side of the body.

ALL ABOUT MIGRAINE

predict the risk of migraine for any given pregnancy. Migraine is such a multifactorial disease that even if we are successful in teasing apart much of the science, we may still not be able to make predictions.

9. What are the different types of migraines?

Migraines are diagnosed like any other medical problem: Doctors use their experience and guidelines to formulate diagnoses. Many people suffer from migraines for years and have never been formally diagnosed. While you may be able to self-diagnose your migraines using books such as this one and resources now easily obtained over the Internet, nothing replaces face-to-face contact with a physician. Medicine does not lend itself to a cookbook approach, no matter how much it appears that this may be the case. You should use the information offered here as a starting point to explore where your headaches may fit in the spectrum of migraine and other headache syndromes. Should you feel that your symptoms are different or not covered, do not hesitate to contact your healthcare provider or a neurologist.

Many people suffer from migraines for years and have never been formally diagnosed.

Over the years neurologists have used varying criteria to diagnose migraine and the other varieties of headaches. In 1988, a group of researchers and clinicians got together and developed ***The International Classification of Headache Disorders***. This classification system has allowed researchers to better study the new agents for the treatment of migraine, and it quickly gained popularity in clinical practice. I tend to use this classification in my practice as much as possible because it provides a uniform set of criteria, allowing me to apply consistency across the patients I see in my clinic. This consistency allows me to get a sense of how medications work with

The International Classification of Headache Disorders

A well-accepted classification used to diagnose headaches. This classification system is also used in research.

the various types of migraine. I always tell my patients that they are not alone in their suffering, yet they remain unique individuals. While this may sound trite, it is true. However, if I am consistent in how I make their diagnosis, I have held constant one of the variables that may affect their response to treatment. This is important because so many other factors will affect how they respond to the treatment plans developed in the office. This classification system also provides an excellent model for teaching new physicians about the diagnosis of migraine. In many ways it is very complementary to the more traditional nomenclature, which makes it even more appealing. The advances in our understanding of migraine have come such a long way in the last decade that the second edition of *The International Classification of Headache Disorders* was recently released. The following paragraphs also include the more traditional terminology that you may encounter as you read more about migraine.

The most common type of migraine is **migraine without aura**. You may also hear this type of migraine called common migraine. This type of migraine must meet specific time criteria and number of episodes. Migraine without aura is accompanied by symptoms such as nausea and vomiting and a desire to sleep in a dark room. The quality of the headache is also important, with migraines generally being throbbing in nature. Migraine without aura frequently accompanies a woman's menstrual cycle. *The International Classification of Headache Disorders* (Second Edition) gives very specific criteria for migraine without aura that many clinicians use in making the diagnosis. These include at least *five* episodes fulfilling the following criteria:

Migraine without aura

A moderately severe to severe headache on one side of the head that is usually accompanied by sensitivity to noise and light, nausea, and vomiting; it is throbbing in nature and lasts anywhere from 4 to 72 hours. Also called common migraine.

- Headache lasting 4 to 72 hours untreated or unsuccessfully treated
- Two of the following: unilateral, pulsating, moderate-to-severe intensity, aggravated by exercise or causing an avoidance of exercise
- At least one of the following: sensitivity to noise and/or light, nausea and/or vomiting
- No other discernible cause for the headache

Migraine with aura

A migraine preceded by flashing lights, visual loss, or other visual or neurological phenomena. Also called classical migraine.

Focal neurological deficit

Numbness, weakness, speech abnormalities, visual changes, difficulties walking, clumsiness, or any other problem with the body that can be attributed to the nervous system.

Predator effect

A type of visual aura similar to the effect seen in the movie Predator, where an object appears to distort the background as though it is being viewed through ground glass.

Scotoma

A dark spot in the field of vision in one eye. May be temporary or permanent.

Less frequent, but an important classification, is **migraine with aura**, also more traditionally referred to as classical migraine. This migraine is characterized by the onset of a **focal neurological deficit** preceding the migraine. This deficit may be visual or physical. With visual auras, symptoms may consist of dark spots, jagged bright lines, or distorted visual phenomenon, which I refer to as the *Predator* **effect** after the movie *Predator*, where the screen was distorted when the Predator was invisible and moving through the scene. This distortion of perception occurs without an actual loss of vision or bright lights and is similar to looking at something through shattered glass. Another type of visual symptom is a **scotoma**, or the actual loss of vision such that it appears as though a hole has been punched out of what one sees. These "holes" may occur in one or both eyes. Other types of auras include numbness on one side of the body and/or face, a sensation of tingling and pins and needles, and difficulty with speech or language.

All of these auras develop over 5 minutes and last up to 60 minutes prior to the onset of a headache that otherwise meets the criteria for migraine without aura. The aura may dissipate as the headache pain comes on, or it may persist throughout the headache. For many migraineurs, on occasion the aura may occur without the headache.

Migraines that are preceded by or accompanied by weakness on one side of the face and/or body are usually considered **sporadic hemiplegic migraines**. The migraines are accompanied by flashing lights or sensory symptoms or speech difficulties and are fully reversible in 24 hours or less. On rare occasions, weakness accompanying migraine may be a sign of a rare hereditary disease called familial hemiplegic migraine (see Question 8). These migraines are similar to sporadic hemiplegic migraine, except that the migraineur has family members afflicted with the same disorder. Both of these migraine types are worked up (process of diagnosis) carefully to rule out other causes for the neurological deficits. It is important to rule out a stroke as the cause of the symptoms, so the work-up may include an MRI or computerized axial tomography (CAT) scan of the brain and its vessels, as well as tests on the heart.

Sporadic hemiplegic migraines

Migraines that are accompanied by a weakness on one side or limb of the body.

Basilar-type migraine is another type of migraine that you may experience. These migraines are characterized by at least two attacks of a migraine with an aura consisting of at least two of the following:

- Slurred speech
- Vertigo (a sensation of the room spinning)
- Tinnitus (ringing in the ears)
- Hyperacusis (noises sounding louder than usual)
- Diplopia (double vision)
- Visual changes in your field of vision near your nasal bridge or outer eye in both eyes
- Ataxia (unsteady gait)
- Decreased level of consciousness
- Tingling simultaneously on both sides of the body

While not as common as other types of migraine, these headaches are often alarming and warrant an evaluation by a neurologist to rule out a stroke or tumor.

10. Are there any complications that I might experience as a result of my migraine?

Chronic migraine

A migraine that occurs 15 or more days per month for 3 months or more.

The complication known as **chronic migraine** is diagnosed when your headaches occur 15 or more days per month for three months or more. This diagnosis is made only when there is no evidence of medication overuse (see Question 29).

Status migrainosis

A migraine that does not respond to the usual treatment and continues for a longer than usual time period. These migraines may last days to over a week and require steroids or narcotics to break the pain.

Another potential complication is **status migrainosis**, defined as a migraine that is of severe intensity lasting longer than 72 hours. Several medications are used to break status migrainosis, including steroids, dihydroergotamine, and/or narcotics. If you frequently suffer from status migrainosis and are not on a prophylactic treatment, this may be a good reason to begin such a regimen.

In recent years, scientists have been studying the long-term effects of migraine on the brain. There is speculation that the long-term risk of stroke may be higher in migraineurs, especially those with aura. The link between dementia and migraine has also been investigated. Some studies have shown that migraine protects against dementia, whereas other studies have shown it is a risk factor for dementia.

11. What if I experience weakness with my migraine that lasts longer than the headache?

Most migraineurs do not experience focal neurological deficits with their headaches. Therefore, it is very frightening to have weakness of the face or limbs before, during, or after a migraine. It is important that you contact your physician immediately if you experience any symptoms with your headache that are of concern to you. Numbness or weakness that is new or that does not resolve is always worrisome. A good rule of thumb is that the first time you experience weakness, numbness, speech difficulties, or visual problems accompanying your migraine, or any headache, you should go to the nearest emergency room to see a doctor. Usually a neurologist will be called to see you to rule out a stroke. Powerful "clot-busting" drugs can be used in acute stroke to reverse the symptoms and prevent further damage to the brain, but these agents must be given within three hours of the onset of symptoms to be effective.

If you have been experiencing these symptoms and they resolve followed by a severe headache, it is likely that they are indicative of migraine with aura or sporadic hemiplegic migraine. Even so, it is very important to rule out more dangerous causes. If you have not seen a doctor, you should have these symptoms checked out by a neurologist. A neurologist may order magnetic resonance imaging (MRI) or computerized axial tomography (CAT) scan to rule out small strokes or other lesions. In addition, your neurologist may request blood work to be done to rule out various causes of strokes and to look for problems that may be genetic. While these causes are unusual, it is important to see a neurologist to confirm that no neurological problem has surfaced.

12. Is every migraine the same?

Cherie's comment:

I remember one of my first migraines, which at the time was caused by a pinched nerve in my neck. The pain radiated from the back of my head into my forehead. I never imagined headache pain could be so severe. With the help of a neck collar and medication, the pain eventually disappeared, but it lasted for several days.

Most migraineurs remember their very first migraine and are able to give a vivid description of what they were doing, the degree of pain they experienced, and how they tried to make it go away. One would think that every migraine would be the same and that every migraine would respond to the same medication or medications; however, this is often not the case. Your headaches should follow a pattern with some degree of variability in their presentation.

Each head-ache may be a bit different in charac-ter, severity, location, and length of time it persists.

Each headache may be a bit different in character, sever-ity, location, and length of time it persists. Medications may work for a period of months to years and then stop being effective. You may find that one medication may work for one headache, only to be ineffective for the next one. The important thing is the degree of differ-ence between the headaches. If there is a large differ-ence between headaches, this may be a danger signal, and you should see a physician immediately. If you are a veteran migraineur, you are probably accustomed to the myriad of forms that your migraines may take and the ways they may descend on you. Some may rudely awaken you at night, while others creep up slowly and inevitably during the course of a stressful day. Many of my patients tell me that they feel a migraine "lurking in the back-ground" before they even feel the pain. This may be the premonitory period described in Question 13 and is the time for many patients to start treating an episode. Still other patients describe episodes of low-level pain that are different from their tension headaches and could blos-som with the right trigger into a full-blown attack.

I spend a great deal of time simply listening to my patients tell me their migraine stories, and most of them tell me about their struggle with a monster called migraine. This monster has many different faces and behaviors. As long as you trust your instincts and follow some basic rules outlined in Question 17 about dangerous headaches, your biggest problem with this aspect of migraine will be finding the best treatment for any given episode.

13. How does migraine differ from other headache types?

Cherie's comment:

The migraines I have experienced for the past several years are all similar in nature. I can't say that I have ever had an "aura" prior to a migraine event, but the headaches usually start on the right side of my head (temple). If I can catch it in time, and if the migraine is not one of the more severe headaches that I've had, then usually something like Tylenol® [acetaminophen] will relieve the pain. However, on occasion I have had serious breakthrough migraines where the pressure is so intense that I can only stay in bed, where it must be quiet and dark. Sometimes the pain will travel from the right temple to the back of my head and into my neck, making my pillow feel like it is as hard as a rock. There are times when I have a migraine, and I can actually see it in my face when I look in the mirror. It can sometimes take almost two days for my serious migraines to completely dissipate. And once they are gone, I am usually left with a feeling of vulnerability where I almost feel as though another headache is lurking around the corner just waiting for me. I simply feel completely and utterly drained of every ounce of energy.

In general, migraine tends to be moderately to severely painful, on one side of the head or the other (often referred to as **unilateral**), throbbing or pulsating (felt in rhythm with your heartbeat), and of such a nature that avoidance of light or noise makes you feel better.

Unilateral

Occurring on one side only.

25

Often nausea and/or vomiting are present, and sometimes vomiting makes the headache feel better. Sleep may make the migraine feel better, and exercise may make the headache worse. If you are a migraine sufferer, these symptoms will sound very familiar to you. You may experience some or all of these symptoms depending on the particular headache, and the severity of the headache may vary, but the migraine headache is generally more painful than other common types of headaches. The exception is when a headache is sudden and severe and the most painful you have ever experienced. As discussed in Question 17, this may be a **dangerous headache**, and you should seek medical attention immediately.

Many times migraines also have **premonitory symptoms**, or a constellation of symptoms preceding the headache. These symptoms tend to warn of an impending migraine and are often useful to the veteran migraineur as a signal to initiate treatment. Such symptoms may consist of listlessness, fatigue, pallor, yawning, and even sensitivity to light and vague nausea.

Migraine tends to occur in lockstep with the menstrual cycle in women. This is unusual for any other type of headache, including **tension-type headaches**. In fact, tension-type headaches tend to occur frequently throughout the month, whereas migraine tends to occur infrequently in comparison.

I often tell my residents and medical students that the diagnosis of migraine and headaches is straightforward if they follow *The International Classification of Headache Disorders* and trust their instincts. In general, it is safe to say that common things occur commonly and that most patients will have either tension-type headaches or migraines, or both.

Dangerous headache

A headache that is not typical for an individual and may be a harbinger of a potentially life-threatening process. All headaches thought to be dangerous should be evaluated or treated.

Premonitory symptoms

Signs of an impending migraine.

Tension headaches

Headaches that are bilateral, pressing, and of mild to moderate severity. Often occur in people who also have migraines.

14. I was told that I have tension headaches as well as migraine headaches. What is the difference, and how do I tell one from the other?

Max's comment:

I have both migraines and "normal" headaches. The migraines last from 24 to 36 hours if they are not treated. Sometimes I can't tell the difference between the two types of headaches, but if I take Tylenol® and it's a "normal" headache, the pain goes away. It's frustrating that sometimes I take Tylenol® only to find that it's really a migraine and I have to take my prescribed medications to relieve the headache.

It is very common for tension headache and migraine headache to occur in the same person. Tension-type headaches are usually bilateral and pressing, as opposed to unilateral and throbbing, and only of mild-to-moderate severity, as opposed to moderate-to-severe pain. They do not worsen with physical activity. According to *The International Classification of Headache Disorders*, they may be accompanied occasionally by sensitivity to light or noise, but they are not accompanied by nausea and vomiting. Tension-type headaches usually occur more frequently than migraine and last for shorter periods of time. They also respond to milder medications, such as acetaminophen or aspirin, or go away on their own.

It is very common for tension headache and migraine headache to occur in the same person.

Because tension-type headaches often occur in people with migraine, it is important to distinguish between the two. If the symptoms of a tension headache are misinterpreted for a migraine and the incorrect medications are taken, a cyclical problem of taking excess medication for more headaches may occur, leading to the medication overuse headaches described in Question 29.

Many neurologists and patients find that using a journal or diary to track their headaches, the symptoms that accompany them, and the medications or treatment approaches that relieve them assists in differentiating between the two headache types.

In my practice, I simply ask patients how many types of headache they have. If the patient has experienced intermittent severe migraine headaches or bad headaches three to four times per month, generally only one type of headache is reported. Those who experience severe headaches interspersed among milder headaches report that they experience two types of headache. It is rare that patients experience three types of headache. If you have tension headache and migraine headache and begin experiencing a new type of headache, it may be time to see a neurologist.

Tension-type headache also may occur infrequently and may be confused with migraine without aura. Once again, the general rule of thumb is that a tension-type headache differs in the quality of the pain, the length of time it persists, its associated symptoms, and its severity. Episodic tension-type headaches also may resolve on their own or with over-the-counter medications, and their treatment often does not require the input of a physician.

Cluster headache

A headache type that occurs primarily in men, characterized by severe pain lasting usually about 45 minutes, accompanied by nasal discharge and pain localized around or behind the eye. Headache episodes cluster temporally, with episodes lasting several months and headache-free periods interspersed.

15. What is a "cluster" headache? Is this a type of migraine?

Many types of headache exist. A cousin of the migraine headache is the **cluster headache**, which is severely painful and often localized on one side of the head. However, this is where the similarities between the two types of headaches tend to end.

Men are three times more likely than women to have cluster headache. It has been noted, however, that recently more women have been diagnosed with this disorder. The "cluster" in cluster headache refers to a temporal clustering of the headaches. Sufferers report bouts of headache every night for three to four months with intervening periods lasting months to years that are pain free. Headache then recurs in the same pattern.

Triggers of cluster headache are well known and include heavy cigarette smoking, alcohol, and erratic sleep patterns. Jet lag and strong odors have also been reported to bring on cluster headache in some individuals with the disorder. These triggers seem to be problematic only during a cluster, however—they do not set off headaches during the intervening quiescent headache-free periods.

Cluster headache pain is localized in the eye area and is often accompanied by tearing and a runny nose. The pain is very intense and lasts for approximately 45 to 90 minutes, although it may go on for hours. This is dissimilar to a migraine, which usually is moderate to severely painful (although a migraine may on occasion be intensely painful) and usually lasts hours to days. Unlike persons with a migraine, individuals with a cluster headache are restless and may become agitated, even to the point of pounding their head against the wall to distract them from the pain. Sufferers may also perform calisthenics or other exercises to distract themselves from the pain—something a typical migraineur could not tolerate.

The mainstay of acute cluster headache treatment is 100% oxygen, which is usually administered in the emergency room during an acute attack. Chronic sufferers may have an oxygen tank ordered for home use by their physician so that it is available in the event of an attack. Triptans are used as an acute treatment with good results and dihydro-ergotamines are also effective (although these two types of medicines must not be used within 24 hours of each other). Because most of these patients live in fear of their next cluster and because headaches can occur daily during an attack, prevention is a very important component of treatment of cluster headaches. One medication that is a particular favorite of neurologists is verapamil, a widely used **blood pressure medication** in the calcium-channel blocker family that has been found to be effective in treating cluster headache. You may be placed on very high doses of this medicine to treat your cluster headache, and you should discuss the risk–benefit trade-off of using these dosages to treat your headaches. Other medications prescribed for cluster headaches include anticonvulsants, steroids, and ergotamines. The latter two are recommended only during a cluster, but not for long-term prevention.

Blood pressure medication

Medicine used to control blood pressure as well as to prevent migraines.

16. Is there a possibility that my headaches are not migraines, but rather are due to a brain tumor?

This is one of the most commonly held beliefs about headaches. Individuals who have suffered for long periods with their headaches may truly believe they have a **brain tumor** or other life-threatening lesion. The prevalence of significant **intracranial lesions** in a person with a diagnosis of migraine and a normal neurological examination is only 0.2%. Given the rarity of this condition, it is highly unlikely that you are harboring a dangerous lesion in your brain that is causing your headaches.

It may be helpful to explore why you are fearful. Do you have a family history of brain tumors? If so, this may be reason enough to have an MRI with contrast or CAT

Brain tumor

Tumors of the brain may be malignant or benign. The most common brain tumor is slow growing and benign and occurs more frequently in women. Many times these tumors cause no problems. Other, more aggressive tumors are much rarer.

Intracranial lesions

Masses, tumors, abnormal blood vessels, blood clots, or other abnormalities located in the brain.

scan, as some tumors may be inherited. You should be sure to tell your physician about this part of your family history. Did someone in your family or circle of friends have a tumor? It might help to compare your history to theirs. When patients of mine take this step, they often find that the only thing they have in common is the headache. Everything else is dissimilar, including the characteristics of their headache.

It is not unusual to be frightened of an illness that strikes down others close to us, or even those we read about. This is why it is important to have regular medical exams, engage in preventive medicine precautions, and work with your physician to understand your fears and concerns. What you should not do is leave the doctor's office without having expressed your fears or worries. In the case of headache, suppressing your concerns is counterproductive because it can lead to further stress and more headaches. Remember, it is okay to be afraid. It is not okay to live with this fear in silence. Regardless of the physician's response, it is often very helpful to verbalize your fears.

It is okay to be afraid. It is not okay to live with this fear in silence.

Which symptoms may be indicative of a tumor? Seizures; confusion; changes in behavior; weakness and numbness on one part of your body; difficulties with vision, smell, speech, or swallowing; nausea and vomiting; and, of course, headaches are some of the symptoms experienced by patients with brain tumors. Headaches that accompany brain tumors are sometimes worse in the morning (although this can be seen with migraine as well). Because we all experience many of these symptoms at one point or another for brief periods of time, the doctor's examination will determine whether the symptoms are significant. Some studies have shown that for people who are not headache sufferers, headache is the presenting and only symptom of a tumor less than 10% of the time. For those who are headache sufferers, a visit to the physician is always warranted when a normal headache pattern worsens, when headaches cease to respond to usual medication regimens, or when symptoms are otherwise worrisome.

17. Are there headaches that are dangerous?

While any headache could potentially be dangerous, it is helpful to understand the spectrum of dangerous headaches. In general, most physicians will keep an eye out for alarming signs and symptoms. You also should be aware of these symptoms and seek medical care if you experience any of them. Conversely, remember that if you are *not* experiencing these signs or symptoms, there is a very high likelihood that you are not experiencing a dangerous headache. Here are some of the **danger signals**:

Headache danger signals

Symptoms and signs that may signal ominous etiologies of a headache. If you experience these types of symptoms, go to an emergency room or contact your physician.

- The worst headache of your life
- Loss of consciousness with onset of a headache
- *Sudden* severe headache that peaks within minutes
- Headache associated with a fever of 101°F or greater, stiff neck, and/or chills
- Headache associated with confused thinking
- Headache following trauma
- Headache associated with new focal neurological deficits (such as the loss of localized muscle control, numbness, weakness, or difficulties with speech)
- Headache in a person with cancer, HIV, or other medical disease that might affect the brain
- Significant worsening or change in pattern of headache in a migraineur or other chronic headache sufferer

The most ominous of the danger signals is the statement, "This is the worst headache of my life." Using it as a guide for diagnosis is tricky, however, because it may be tempting to overstate your predicament in your desperation to obtain pain relief from a migraine. Physicians will take a complaint of the "worst headache of my life" very seriously and may begin a very aggressive work-up to rule out bleeding in your brain. The work-up itself is not without some risks, so it behooves you to use this phrase only when it is accurate. If what you really mean is that you are having your typical migraine and it is wearing you down, and that you are feeling frustrated and at your wit's end, then convey that message to your doctor.

Physicians will take a complaint of the "worst headache of my life" very seriously.

A very severe headache that is abrupt in onset (occurs over a matter of seconds), especially if it is associated with loss of consciousness and/or numbness or weakness or speech difficulties, may be due to a ruptured aneurysm or a stroke, and you should see a doctor immediately. Usually these headaches are so sudden and severe that bystanders or family members call 911. If you are a migraineur and you experience this type of headache, it may not be a migraine, and you should go to your nearest emergency room and call your personal physician. At the hospital you will have a neurological examination, a computed tomography scan (often called a CT scan or CAT scan) and perhaps an MRI, and, if necessary, a **lumbar puncture**. The lumbar puncture will allow the physician to evaluate the fluid that bathes your brain and spinal cord for blood. If a blood vessel has ruptured, blood will appear in that fluid. If you have had a bleed, this fact should show up on the brain scans. If your examination and brain scans are negative, you may be given another diagnosis and tested for other medical problems. If the lumbar puncture is positive,

Lumbar puncture

A procedure done to obtain spinal fluid by inserting a needle into the base of the spine between vertebrae (also known as a spinal tap). The needle does not touch the spinal cord because it is below the level of the spinal cord, or nerves, but only extracts fluid. This fluid is then sent to a lab for analysis.

a neurosurgeon will be called and further tests will be done to determine the location of the aneurysm and the best approach to repair it.

A severe headache that is accompanied by fever greater than 101°F, stiff neck, and/or chills should be evaluated by a physician. The most likely reason for this constellation of symptoms is the common infection known as viral meningitis, but bacterial meningitis and more serious viral infections must be considered. After you arrive at the hospital, blood work including blood cultures will probably be done, followed by a neurological examination, CAT scan of the brain, and possibly a lumbar puncture. If an infection is found, medications may be started and a short hospital stay may be necessary to monitor your fever, blood pressure, and blood cell counts.

Trauma is another common cause of headache in our society. A severe headache associated with trauma of any kind should be evaluated by a physician or emergency department. You should see a physician as soon as you begin experiencing a severe headache. *Do not wait!* The doctors will evaluate you for a concussion and bleeding in your brain by asking you questions, examining you, and doing a CAT scan. This is one time where a CAT scan—not an MRI—is generally the preferred test because blood and fractures can often be seen more clearly on a CAT scan. After being evaluated, if you are sent home, you will probably be given an instruction sheet listing the symptoms to watch out for over the next 24 to 72 hours and, what to do should they occur. If the doctors find blood or a fracture, you may be kept in the hospital overnight for observation and be evaluated by a neurosurgeon. While these measures may sound very alarming to the layperson, trauma injuries are the "bread and butter" of most emergency rooms.

Strokes are another potentially dangerous cause of headaches. Usually strokes are accompanied by focal neurological deficits such as numbness, weakness, or speech difficulties. Headache may be the sole symptom, but this is unusual, especially in a young adult. If you have risk factors for stroke such as hypertension, diabetes, high cholesterol levels, a history of smoking, or a previous stroke, and you experience a new headache that is unusual for you, you should contact your physician or go to the nearest emergency room if you believe you are having a stroke.

Headaches in the setting of a medical disease that may have associated neurological complications may be potentially dangerous. Certain cancers may metastasize to the brain, and certain infections might go to the brain in the person with HIV infection or acquired immune deficiency syndrome (AIDS). If you experience a headache and also have a medical problem, contact your physician to discuss whether the headache may be due to medications, a complication of your medical problem, or a primary headache disorder. Your doctor may refer you to a neurologist to help sort matters out.

If you notice a change in your pattern of headaches or you notice that your headaches are worsening, this change may be a danger signal. Having migraines does not protect you from having other disorders of the brain. If you notice a change that is sustained and troubling, speak with your physician, especially if you have been treating your migraines with over-the-counter medications. This may be a good time to have a complete medical and/or neurological evaluation.

If you notice a change in your headache pattern that is sustained and troubling, speak with your physician.

While not exactly a danger signal per se, new-onset headache in a person older than age 45 or 50 usually gives most clinicians pause. Migraine and tension headache rarely begin in later life, leaving the more unusual headache disorders as the culprits. For this reason, many primary care physicians will refer patients in this age range to neurologists for evaluation, and many people will also go to a neurologist directly for evaluation and reassurance.

PART TWO

Treatment and the Doctor's Visit

What type of pharmacological approaches do physicians use in the treatment of migraine?

What are some of the medications my doctor might recommend or prescribe?

What if none of my usual migraine treatments work? At what point do I go to the emergency room?

More . . .

18. What type of pharmacological approaches do physicians use in the treatment of migraine?

Stepwise approach

Method of treating migraine that entails starting with first-line, low-strength medicines, and increasing to stronger and more specific drugs until pain relief is achieved.

The majority of clinicians follow one of two general pharmacological approaches to the treatment of migraine in their patients. The first is the **stepwise approach**. In this approach the physician starts with a class of medications and changes the strength and/or perhaps the specificity of medicine if your pain does not improve. An example of this type of approach would be to start with acetaminophen if your headaches sound mild in nature and then increase the strength of the treatment to nonsteroidal anti-inflammatory drugs (NSAIDs) if necessary. Even stronger medications will be used until pain relief is achieved.

Stratified approach

Method of treating migraine that entails starting with the most appropriate medication based on the patient's symptoms, lifestyle, and resources.

Although the stepwise approach may work for some people, an increasingly preferable approach is the **stratified approach**, which emphasizes the selection of a specific medication after taking multiple issues into consideration. These factors may include the type of headache you have, its severity, your lifestyle, the potential side effects of the medication, your resources, and your cultural background. This approach is often preferred because it saves time and is very patient focused. It also takes into account the fundamental goals of acute migraine management. These goals have been nicely defined in the *Evidence-Based Guidelines for Migraine Headache in the Primary Care Setting: Pharmacologic Management of Acute Attacks*, which can be found on the website of the American Academy of Neurology. They are reproduced here with permission:

- Treat attacks rapidly and consistently without recurrence.
- Restore the patient's ability to function.

- Minimize the use of backup and rescue medications.
- Optimize self-care, and reduce subsequent use of resources.
- Be cost-effective for overall management.
- Have minimal or no side effects.

For the stratified approach to be successful, you must share enough information with the physician so that the appropriate medication or medications may be selected. The physician may also give you several types of medications to use in specific circumstances, so that you have various options to try depending on the type and severity of your migraine. An example of this approach would be to give you one of the triptans to relieve your migraine immediately rather than seeing if a milder agent will be effective.

Finally, keep in mind that the goal of treatment is a reduction in headache frequency and severity and an increase in your control over your migraines. Research studies often specify a 50% reduction in number of headaches as a measure of successful treatment. Therefore, you should adjust your expectations accordingly.

19. What are some of the medications my doctor might recommend or prescribe?

Table 1 gives short descriptions of many of the specific medications used to treat migraine.

Generally speaking, nonprescription medications used to treat individual episodes include simple **analgesics**, used for their pain relief properties, and **nonsteroidal anti-inflammatory drugs (NSAIDs)**, used for their anti-inflammatory effects and analgesic properties. Prescription medications are also used to treat individual

Analgesics
Pain-relieving medications.

Nonsteroidal anti-inflammatory drug (NSAID)
Medication used to abort migraine. Also used in many other pain syndromes where inflammation may be felt to play a role.

Table 1 Medications used to treat or prevent migraines.

Type of Medicine	Generic	Trade	Dosages	Indication: Episodic or Prevention	Evidence	Side Effects
Nonprescription						
Analgesics	Acetaminophen	Tylenol®	650–1300 mg every 4–6 hrs	Episodic	+	Very well tolerated in most people
	Aspirin	Bayer®	650–1300 mg every 4–6 hrs	Episodic	+++	Gastrointestinal irritation and/or bleeding; coated varieties may lessen these effects
	Aspirin with caffeine, aspirin with caffeine and acetaminophen	Excedrin Migraine®	2 tablets every 4–6 hrs	Episodic	+++	
NSAIDs—non-steroidal anti-inflammatory drugs	Naproxen sodium	Aleve®, Naprosyn®	275–550 mg every 6–8 hrs	Episodic	+++	Gastrointestinal irritation and/or bleeding; taking these medications with meals or crackers may lessen these effects
	Ibuprofen	Motrin®	400–800 mg every 6–8 hrs	Episodic	+++	Possible cardiac ischemia
Prescription						
NSAIDs—non-steroidal anti-inflammatory drugs	Celecoxib	Celebrex®	100 mg–200 mg once or twice per day	Episodic	+	Possible stroke or cardiac ischemia with prolonged use
Combination medications (other than ergotamines)	Butalbital/acetaminophen/ caffeine	Fioricet®, Esgic®	1–2 tablets every 4 hrs	Episodic	+	Drowsiness (note that drowsiness may be offset if the preparation contains caffeine) and/or rash. Do not use if you have an allergy to barbiturates.
	Butalbital/acetaminophen	Phrenilin®	1–2 tablets every 4 hrs	Episodic	+	

Category	Generic	Brand	Dose	Type	Effectiveness	Side effects
	Isometheptene/acetaminophen/dichloralphenzone	Midrin®	2 capsules at headache onset then 1 tablet every ½ hr as needed up to 3 doses	Episodic	+++	Isometeptene: dizziness, rash
	Sumatriptan/naproxen sodium	Treximet®	1 tablet at headache onset; repeat at 2 hrs as needed; no more than 2 doses in 24 hours	Episodic	+++	Same as triptans and NSAIDS
Antinauseants	Metaclopramide	Reglan®	10 mg at headache or nausea onset	Episodic	+++	Restlessness, muscle spasms, dizziness, sedation
	Prochlorperazine	Compazine®	1 suppository OR 25 mg by mouth at headache or nausea onset	Episodic	+++	
Ergotamine preparations	Ergotamine tartrate/caffeine	Cafergot®	1–2 mg by mouth or suppository repeated once as needed; not to be repeated more than 3 times per week	Episodic	++	Ergotamine preparations: diarrhea, muscle cramps; nausea, tingling in the extremities
	Dihydroergotamine mesylate	Migranal®	2 mg nasally one time at headache onset	Episodic	+++	
Triptans	Almotriptan malate	Axert®	6.25 mg and 12.5 mg tablets	Episodic	+++	All Triptans: "Weird" sensations such as warmth and pressure in throat and upper chest or other parts of the body; tingling in extremities; sleepiness, dizziness, and nausea. A bad taste may be experienced with nasal preparations and injection site reactions may be experienced with subcutaneous injections.
	Eletriptan hydrobromide	Relpax®	20mg, 40mg tablets	Episodic	+++	
	Frovatriptan succinate	Frova®	2.5 mg tablets	Episodic/Prevention	+++	
	Naratriptan hydrochloride	Amerge®	1mg, 2.5 mg tablets	Episodic/Prevention	+++	

(continues)

Table 1 Medications used to treat or prevent migraines (continued).

Type of Medicine	Generic	Trade	Dosages	Indication: Episodic or Prevention	Evidence	Side Effects
Triptans (continued)	Rizatriptan benzoate	Maxalt®	5 mg, 10 mg tablets; MLT 10 mg orally disintegrating tablets	Episodic	+++	
	Sumatriptan succinate	Imitrex®	25 mg, 50 mg, 100 mg rapid dispersion tablets (dissolve rapidly in the stomach); 20 mg intranasal; 6 mg subcutaneous injection	Episodic	+++	
	Zolmitriptan	Zomig®	5 mg; ZMT 2.5 mg orally disintegrating tablets; 5 mg intranasal	Episodic	+++	
Steroids	Prednisone	various	Taper over 7 days (60 mg decreasing by 10 mg per day)	Episodic	+++	Gastric irritation, elated mood, increased blood pressure, increased blood sugar in diabetics
	Methylprednisolone	Medrol Dose Pak®	Prepackaged steroid taper	Episodic	+++	
	Dexamethasone	Decadron®	8 to 12 mg to break headache episode	Episodic	+++	
Narcotics	Butorphanol nasal spray	Stadol®	1 spray at headache onset	Episodic	+++	Sedation, nausea, constipation, itching
	Morphine	MS Contin®	15 to 30 mg tablets	Episodic		
Anti-convulsants	Divalproex sodium	Depakote®	1250 to 2400 mg per day in divided doses	Prevention	+++	Drowsiness, hair loss, tremor, weight-gain, and nausea
	Gabapentin	Neurontin®	900 to 2400 mg per day in divided doses	Prevention	+++	Dizziness, unsteadiness, lethargy

Class	Generic	Brand	Dose	Use	Rating	Side effects
	Topiramate	Topamax®	100 to 400 mg per day in divided doses	Prevention	+++	Fatigue, dizziness, unsteadiness, tingling in the fingers, nervousness, word finding difficulties, weight loss, kidney stones—one must drink 8 ten-ounce glasses of water per day while on this medicine
	Zonisamide	Zonegran®	100 to 300 mg per day in divided doses	Prevention	+++	Abdominal pain; anxiety; difficulty with memory; dizziness; double vision; loss of appetite; nausea
Antidepressants	Amitriptyline	Elavil®	10 to 100 mg per day	Prevention	+++	Drowsiness, dry mouth, weight gain, urinary retention, dizziness, rhythm problems with the heart
	Nortriptyline	Pamelor®	10 to 100 mg per day	Prevention	+++	Similar to amytriptyline but milder
	Phenelzine	Nardil®	15 mg three times a day	Prevention	++	Discomfort, malaise, tremors, dizziness on standing up
	Venlafaxine	Effexor®	37.5 to 75 mg per day	Prevention	+++	Constipation, dizziness, dry mouth, insomnia, nausea, nervousness, sleepiness, sweating, and weakness
Blood pressure medicines	Propranolol	Inderal®	40 to 240 mg per day	Prevention	+++	Slow heart beat, depression, tiredness, sexual dysfunction, memory problems, worsening asthma, difficulty appreciating symptoms of hypoglycemia in diabetes
	Nadolol	Corgard®	20 to 240 mg per day	Prevention	+++	
	Atenolol	Tenormin®	50 to 150 mg per day	Prevention	+++	
	Timolol	Blocadren®	10 to 20 mg per day	Prevention	+++	

(continues)

43

Table 1 Medications used to treat or prevent migraines (continued).

Type of Medicine	Generic	Trade	Dosages	Indication: Episodic or Prevention	Evidence	Side Effects
Blood pressure medicines (continued)	Verapamil	Calan®	180 to 320 mg per day (much higher doses may be used in cluster headache)	Prevention	+++	Swelling of the ankles, dizziness, and nausea
Others	Riboflavin (Vitamin B$_2$)	Various	400 mg per day	Prevention	++	Orange discoloration of urine and stool
	Magnesium	Various	400 to 500 mg per day	Prevention	++	Gastrointestinal upset; diarrhea
	Petasites hybridus extract, aka butter burr	Petadolex®		Prevention	++	None
	Tanacetum parthenium, aka bachelor's buttons, Feverfew			Prevention	++	Mouth sores, dermatitis, may thin blood and lead to bleeding and/or bruising
	Coenzyme Q10			Prevention		

episodes; these agents include NSAIDs known as Cox-2 inhibitors, probably better known for their effectiveness against arthritis (celecoxib [Celebrex®]), and combination drugs. Combination drugs take advantage of multiple mechanisms for aborting migraine. Antinauseants—medicines that relieve the nausea associated with migraine—have been shown to relieve the pain of migraine as well. **Ergotamine** preparations are potent **vasoconstrictors** that compress the blood vessels. Triptans are active at specific brain receptors and are effective vasoconstrictors. Maximum dosages per day should be followed carefully for the triptans and, in general, no more than three triptan treatments should be used per week to avoid medication overuse headaches (see also Question 20 on triptans). Ergotamines and triptans should never be used within 24 hours of each other.

Severe bouts of migraine, called status migrainosis, may be treated with steroids, which are powerful anti-inflammatory agents. Narcotics such as butorphanol nasal spray or morphine may be used in severe cases, as they are potent painkillers.

Prescription medications are also used to prevent episodes of migraine. **Antiepileptic medications** that stabilize the membranes of neurons, making them less susceptible to triggers, are sometimes used for this purpose. Note that your physician may start you at lower doses of these drugs than noted in Table 1 to determine your tolerance for side effects and efficacy. Also keep in mind that these medications may take up to 2 to 4 weeks to work. **Antidepressant medications**, blood pressure medications (especially the beta blockers), vitamins such as **riboflavin** (vitamin B$_2$), and minerals such as magnesium are sometimes used for prevention of migraines as well.

TREATMENT AND THE DOCTOR'S VISIT

Ergotamine

Medicine that is a potent constrictor of blood vessels and that is used to abort migraine attacks.

Vasoconstrictor

A medicine that causes blood vessels to constrict.

Antiepileptic medications

Medications that work to prevent seizures, stabilize moods, and prevent pain.

Antidepressant medications

Medications that work to either enhance or alter chemicals in the brain. They work to improve mood as well as prevent pain.

Riboflavin

Vitamin B$_2$. This vitamin has been found useful in decreasing the frequency and number of days of migraine attacks if taken regularly in doses of 400 mg.

The list in Table 1 is not exhaustive, but it covers most of the drugs for which studies support their use in migraine, those for which there are studies ongoing, and those that are commonly used by neurologists for migraine. Your physician may suggest other agents that he or she has found useful in the treatment or prevention of migraine. In general, these medications will fall into one of the general classes of medicines listed.

20. What are triptans?

Triptans are now the gold standard in the acute treatment of migraine. This class of medications was developed to very specifically intervene in the neurochemical cascade that causes the pain of a migraine. These drugs work at the serotonin receptor level, are generally well tolerated, and have played such a major role in treatment of migraine that they have revolutionized migraine management. Prior to the use of these drugs, many patients were unable to function or get relief from their pain. Since the release of the first triptan, sumatriptan, in the early 1990s, many migraineurs have been able to awaken with a severe migraine, take a triptan, and go off to work an hour later, pain free. Few other areas of medicine can boast such a dramatic advance in treatment as well as in the quality of life of patients.

Since the development of the first triptan, several other members of this drug class have been introduced. Although the triptans differ somewhat on a chemical basis, you should be aware of the similarities and differences that will be the most important to you, as the consumer, should your doctor prescribe one or more of these medications. All of the triptans basically are active at the serotonin receptor and have the best effect the earlier they are taken in the migraine episode. Nevertheless, if you take a triptan later in an episode, you might still achieve very good pain relief. Many patients do not take their triptan to alleviate pain simply because they think that if they do not take it early, it will not work. In reality, while this medication may not work as well for some people later in an attack, it is still better to have some pain relief than to suffer needlessly with the discomfort of a migraine.

Triptans have a tendency to act on vessel walls, so there is some risk of spasm of the heart vessels with their use. For this reason, your doctor will ask you questions about your personal and family history of coronary disease and, if you are older than a certain age, may not prescribe the drug without first doing an appropriate cardiac work-up. Worries about potential cardiac side effects are probably one of the biggest reasons for not prescribing triptans to some patients. However, the risk is less than 1 in 1 million.

All triptans cause an interesting phenomenon referred to as the **triptan effect**. Generally it is described as a warmth or fullness in the chest and neck, a slight light-headedness, tingling in the arms and legs, vague nausea, and sleepiness. Some patients simply refer to it as feeling "strange" or "weird" for 15 or 20 minutes as the medicine starts to take effect. The triptan effect may occur at varying times from the time the dose is taken depending on the brand. It is not particularly pleasant, but like most things you are warned about in advance, it is not as bad when you know what to expect.

Triptan effect

Sensation of warmth, fullness in the throat, tingling in the arms and legs, dizziness, and nausea felt a short while after taking a triptan preparation.

No more than two to three doses of triptans should be taken in a 24-hour period depending on the triptan, and you should avoid taking triptans more than three days per week to decrease the risk of medication overuse headaches. You also should not take these medications if you are taking any cafergot-containing medications or if you are taking a monoamine oxidase (MAO) inhibitor such as phenelzine (Nardil®).

Triptans are expensive medications. They may average anywhere from $8 to $25 per dose depending on the formulation. Some insurance companies restrict which one you may use, generally based on cost concerns. If you need a triptan that is not covered by your insurance, most physicians will work with you to obtain approval. Be sure to let your physician know whether your insurance has any pharmacy restrictions, and do not delay asking for a letter if it is needed to justify the need for triptans. You must advocate for yourself and ask your physician to work with you. The more information your doctor has regarding the specifics of your plan, the better. This will be a real time saver for everyone.

Advocate for yourself and ask your physician to work with you.

The differences between the triptans tend to revolve around the mode of administration or formulation (nasal inhalation, pill, melting wafer, **subcutaneous injection**) and the rapidity of onset of action (which is related to the formulation).

Subcutaneous injection

Injection of medication given directly below the skin.

Sumatriptan (Imitrex®) is the only brand that comes as a subcutaneous injection. This injection is often used in emergency rooms and by patients who cannot tolerate anything by mouth during an attack and require immediate relief. The downsides of this medication are its high cost per dose, the irritation it produces at the injection site, its low desirability among those who are afraid of giving themselves injections, and a more dramatic triptan effect (because this formulation works faster, the triptan effect comes on more quickly and is a bit more intense). The effectiveness of the medicine also does not last as long if your migraine tends to last a long time.

Sumatriptan and zolmitriptan both have nasal forms that can be used by those who are unable to take pills due to nausea. Their downsides are a slightly unpleasant taste in the back of the throat, burning of the nasal tissues in some people, and a higher cost than pills.

Frovatriptan and naratriptan are pills with a slower onset of action; they last somewhat longer and have a milder triptan effect, but they may not be as effective for very severe headaches. However, these preparations are gaining significant popularity with many patients and headache specialists in the treatment of menstrual migraine and in the prevention of migraine prior to activities known to trigger a migraine. You can see how beneficial this ability might be if you have a special event coming up where you wish to wear a favorite perfume that sets off a migraine or eat a special food that sometimes triggers a migraine.

Almotriptan, eletriptan, rizatriptan, sumatriptan, and zolmitriptan are pills with a more rapid onset of action, triptan effect, and effective migraine relief. Rizatriptan and zolmitriptan also come in rapidly dissolving wafers that may be easier to take for those people who have nausea and find it difficult to swallow pills or who vomit due to their migraine. Imitrex® tablets now are formulated to be rapidly dispersing in the stomach so that they dissolve more easily.

The newest addition to the triptan armamentarium is a medication that combines sumatriptan with naproxyn sodium, called Treximet™. This combination of a triptan and an NSAID in one pill simultaneously uses two different mechanisms of migraine treatment. In studies of Treximet™, the combination worked better in reducing the pain and associated symptoms of migraine than **placebo**, sumatriptan alone, or naproxyn sodium alone. There is no evidence that this combination therapy has more side effects than either medication alone. Nevertheless, as with all new medications, you should be sure to discuss common side effects with your physician if you are prescribed Treximet™.

As you might imagine, pharmaceutical companies continue to develop even better formulations of triptans. When you consider the vast number of people in our society with migraine, it is clear that there is a huge market for these drugs. It is important that you keep up with the latest advances in drug therapy. One of the best ways to do so is through national organizations such as ACHE and the National Headache Foundation (see the Appendix).

21. What are some of the medication combinations my doctor might prescribe?

Physicians generally use two types of medications in the treatment of migraine: **abortive medications** and **prophylactic medications**.

Abortive medications are used to stop an attack once it has started. Medicines in this category include simple analgesics, combination analgesics containing butalbital/acetaminophen/caffeine, nonsteroidal anti-inflammatory drugs (NSAIDs), triptans, ergotamines, antinauseants, steroids, magnesium, and narcotics. These drugs are taken at the first sign of a migraine to abort the attack and may be repeated if necessary. Your physician may give you one or several of these medicines to take either together or in a stepwise fashion if the first

Placebo

An inactive substance given, usually during a research trial, to compare its effect with the actual drug. Many have an effect from placebos due to suggestion, referred to as a placebo effect.

Abortive medications

Medicines used to stop a migraine attack once it has started.

Prophylactic medications

Medications used to prevent migraines and/or decrease the frequency and severity of your migraines. These medicines usually take several weeks to work and are usually used in combination with abortive migraine treatments.

agent does not work (see Question 18 on stratified and stepwise approaches to migraine management). Of all these medicines, the only ones that absolutely may not be taken in combination are triptans and ergotamines. These medications have similar actions and side effects, so they may be dangerous if taken together or within 24 hours of each other. The other medications may be sedating or have some cumulative side effects if taken in combination, so you should read all pharmacy and physician instructions carefully.

Prophylactic medicines are taken to prevent migraine or to decrease their frequency and severity. Prophylactic medicines are generally given in either of the following circumstances:

- You are experiencing migraines more than four times per month.
- You are missing work or not functioning well at work for two days per month.

You also may decide with your physician to take prophylactic medicine if you have focal neurological deficits with your headaches, have medical problems that prohibit the use of effective abortive treatments (such as a heart condition), or simply would rather take medicine daily to avoid attacks. Conversely, you may have many migraines per month and decline prophylactic medicines, preferring instead to take only abortive medicines. Perhaps you do not wish to take daily medicines, you are not that troubled by frequent headaches, your headaches are not consistent enough in frequency to warrant daily medications, or you cannot tolerate the side effects of the prophylactic medicines. In recent years, scientists have begun to study the long-term effects of migraine on the brain. While the evidence is not clear at this point, migraine has been associated with stroke and dementia. Thus prevention of migraines may become important in the prevention of later brain disease. Be sure to discuss these issues thoroughly with your doctor so that you make informed decisions about how you treat your migraines.

Prophylactic medicines include antihypertensives, antidepressants, anticonvulsants, vitamins, magnesium, and herbal supplements. These medicines are usually taken once or twice a day. If they are taken once a day, they are usually taken at night so that any side effects (like sleepiness or dizziness) will be less bothersome. Most of these drugs are safe in combination with the abortive agents; however, you should always check with your pharmacist when picking up your prescriptions.

Medication errors account for a fair amount of medical misadventure in the United States. You can take several steps to protect yourself against medication errors. First, if your physician is handwriting your prescription, be sure that YOU can read it before you leave the office. If you cannot read it, there is no reason to believe that a pharmacist will be able to do so. Next, make sure that you use the same pharmacy to get all your medicines; if you do not, let the pharmacist know which other medications you are taking when you get a new medicine prescription filled. Most pharmacies now use automatic medication interaction checkers—computer programs that check your profile of medications against a new medicine to assure that you will not experience any unsafe interactions among your medicines. Finally, make sure that you received the correct quantity of pills and that you understand all instructions on how to take them before you leave the pharmacy. Pharmacists are always willing and able to answer your questions, and a good relationship with your pharmacist is worth the effort if you ever need to negotiate a refill with a pounding headache!

22. What if none of my usual migraine treatments work? At what point do I go to the emergency room?

Given how common migraine is, very few migraineurs use the emergency room as a resource to gain access to care. That said, there may be times when such a visit is unavoidable. As discussed in Question 17, headaches that are associated with a trip to the emergency department may be life-saving. If you are a migraineur who is experiencing a totally different type of headache that is severe in nature or alarming in any other way, a call to your physician is certainly warranted, as is going to the emergency room if needed. The hope of most patients and their physicians is that visits to the emergency room will not be necessary to break a migraine. Indeed, the vast majority of migraineurs never visit the emergency room. Nevertheless for some people—especially those with very severe migraines—trips to the emergency room may be a fact of life.

It is important to work with your physician to create a plan that addresses the steps you should take if you fail to improve with your medications. Prevention is always the best cure. Failing that, be sure you have maximized the medications that you have at home and have tried all relaxation techniques, been totally sequestered in a dark quiet room, and enlisted family and/or friends to help with child care or chores.

If you are in severe pain and have used all medications at your disposal with no relief, a trip to the emergency room may afford you the opportunity to receive intravenous medications or other combinations of medications that may abort the headache.

If your headache is accompanied by nausea and vomiting to the degree that you cannot take in fluids or any type of nourishment for more than 12 hours, you should consider contacting your physician or going to the emergency room. This is especially true if you have diabetes and take medication (insulin and/or pills) for this condition and/or if you take water pills for high blood pressure.

Remember to plan ahead when you travel and around holidays, as these are times when headaches are often more frequent and more painful. Also, always have medication on hand at home at the bedside, in your purse or wallet, and in your office. Remember to refill medications promptly, and do not discontinue any medications without discussing that move first with your physician. I tell my patients to keep a few doses of their abortive medicines in their bedside table and in their purse or wallet *at all times*. Now that effective medicines to treat migraine pain are available, we want you to have ready access to them (and be sure they are not in your medicine cabinet at home when you are vacationing at the beach!).

If you go to the emergency room, take all of your medications with you, and be sure to tell the physician or nurse all the medications taken in the preceding 24 to 48 hours. After any episode that takes you to the emergency room, call your physician to discuss your medication regimen, the trigger for the particular event, and the treatment you received in the emergency room.

23. Under what circumstances might I be admitted to the hospital for a migraine?

These days it is unlikely that you will be admitted for your migraine. Instead, you will probably be given fluids by vein and medications by vein or injection. One indication for admission is if you are so dehydrated and ill that your **electrolytes** cannot be corrected in the emergency room.

A more likely reason for an admission is related to the reason for your severe migraine. If your migraine is caused by medication overuse (Question 29), you may be admitted to wean you off of the offending medication in a safe and comfortable manner using medications that are not easily administered at home. **Medication overuse headaches** (also referred to as rebound headaches) occur when medications are taken very frequently to control migraine or tension-type headaches. As the medications are cleared from the body by the kidney and liver, and the level of the medicine drops, the headache returns and the migraineur takes more medicine, starting the cycle all over again. If you are unwittingly caught in this vicious cycle and stop the offending medicine abruptly, the resulting headache is often unbearable—so bad that it will drive many migraineurs to the emergency room. I often tell my residents in training that if they see a migraineur in the emergency room with a severe migraine, they should rule out a medication overuse headache after they have considered all of the more dangerous possibilities discussed in Question 17.

It is also possible that you might be electively admitted to the hospital for more intensive treatment of your migraine. Many headache centers will admit patients for treatments that require close monitoring, intravenous

Electrolytes

The substances in the blood that keep the fluids in your body in balance. Extreme sweating, vomiting, and diarrhea may throw your electrolytes out of balance, making you feel weak and unable to function.

Medication overuse headaches

Headaches that occur when medications are used daily.

medication administration, or as part of a multidisciplinary approach to care. Usually this type of approach is reserved for more refractory (difficult) cases, but may be very beneficial if you have not found relief through the usual treatments.

24. Is it safe to take several different kinds of medications for migraine?

Many options for headache relief are available. Sometimes one type of medication does not work, so many physicians will suggest a combination of different medications to treat the actual migraine and/or a regimen that is intended to prevent the migraine altogether. Some patients find that one medication may work for one headache but not for another. All headaches are not the same and may need to be treated differently; therefore, having several medications on hand is a wise idea if your goal is adequate pain relief. It is of paramount importance, however, that you understand what each medication is used for, when and at what intervals you should take it, and which medications may be taken safely. Keeping track of your headaches and the degree of relief achieved with your regimen in a journal or diary is very useful for this purpose.

All headaches are not the same and may need to be treated differently.

Potential interactions among medications, both for headaches and for other medical problems, should be discussed in detail with your physician and your pharmacist. It is particularly important that you use only one pharmacy if you are taking several medications and/or if more than one physician is prescribing medications for you. This consistency assures a reliable tracking of all your medications, leads to automatic checks for interactions between medications when a new medication is added, and allows you the potential for developing a relationship with the pharmacist, which may prove beneficial to your health care.

All of the physicians who prescribe your medicines should be aware of *all* medications that you are taking. It is critical that all of your physicians also know that you are in treatment with other physicians and be aware of how to get in touch with them. Medication errors are a frequent cause of medical problems in the United States, and every hospital and physician office patient-safety program usually includes a medication safety component. Make sure you play your part in this nation-wide effort. Be candid about all the medications you are taking, and update all of your physicians on each visit. Include vitamins and any other substances or interventions, even if you are unsure whether they may be relevant. Often vitamins have side effects and interactions with mainstream medications, and these effects may be dangerous if your prescribing physician is unaware of something that you are taking. Open discussions of risks and benefits are always the answer to preventing medication errors.

Be candid about all the medications you are taking, and update all of your physicians on each visit.

Should you ever feel uncomfortable or coerced without adequate explanations about why a physician is recommending a specific change in medications, you should make every attempt to obtain information in an open and nonconfrontational manner. Should this discussion prove unsuccessful, or should the physician be unwilling to work with you and/or your other physicians, or be disparaging of another physician's approach or plan of care, you may wish to consider changing physicians.

25. Why did my doctor prescribe seizure medicines for my headaches? Are my headaches really epilepsy?

Seizure

Electrical discharges in the brain leading to alterations or loss of consciousness.

Comorbid

Diseases that occur together but are not related to each other.

Urinary incontinence

Involuntary loss of urine due to a neurological cause (e.g., seizures, multiple sclerosis, spinal cord injury), urological causes, gynecological causes, coughing, laughing, and so forth.

Generalized seizures

Seizures during which patients lose consciousness, their limbs jerk, and they often urinate on themselves and bite their tongues.

Complex partial seizures

Seizures that alter an individual's consciousness and may be associated with speech abnormalities and arm movements.

Max's comment:

I had migraines for many years prior to being diagnosed with a seizure disorder. I was in my thirties when I had my first **seizure**. *Originally, I took Dilantin®, but recently switched to Depakote®. Although Depakote® is sometimes prescribed for headaches, it has not altered the frequency or severity of my migraines. The most effective medication that I have found is Zomig®. Supposedly, Zomig® should be taken within a half hour of the headache's onset, but I can take it at any time and it will work.*

Many medications are prescribed for multiple purposes. Medications that are prescribed for epilepsy, for example, have been found to be effective in treating migraine headaches as well. Although epilepsy and migraine are certainly different diseases, some of the chemicals involved with these diseases are the same or similar. In fact, there is some evidence that migraine and epilepsy are often **comorbid**, and they occur together more often than you would expect by chance.

Epilepsy is a disease that usually begins in younger people in their teens or early adulthood. It is manifested by loss of consciousness and shaking of the limbs with tongue biting and **urinary incontinence**—a phenomenon known as **generalized seizures**. Smaller seizures, called **complex partial seizures**, are usually seen with a brief alteration in consciousness, and sometimes involuntary mouth or hand and arm movements. Even though awake, the person is usually not aware of his or her surroundings.

Migraines and seizures are similar in that they are both paroxysmal (intermittently occurring) events in the brain. Because the underlying cause is primarily a disruption in chemical processes, which are similar, the medications used to treat the two conditions are the same, though the dosages used for migraine are often lower than those used in epilepsy. These medications are usually given to prevent migraines and are taken one to three times per day. It is rare that these medications are given to treat an individual headache.

If you are prescribed an anticonvulsant for your migraine, it is important that you understand why that particular medication was chosen and which types of side effects you might experience. One of the commonly used anticonvulsants, divalproex sodium (Depakote®), may require that you have your blood drawn regularly to monitor your liver function and the level of drug in your system.

It is also important that you never stop any of these medications abruptly. Anticonvulsants should be started gradually and stopped gradually. Even if you do not have seizures, abruptly withdrawing from these medications can irritate the brain cells and may cause a seizure.

26. Do vitamins and herbal supplements help in the treatment of migraine?

Alternatives to traditional medications may be beneficial for patients who cannot tolerate the side effects of these medications or in whom the use of these medications may be potentially dangerous owing to their other medical conditions. For this reason, researchers have studied vitamins as potential agents to treat and prevent migraines. There are theoretical bases for certain vitamins being effective agents, the first and foremost being riboflavin (vitamin B$_2$).

Riboflavin is important in the release of energy during metabolism as well as many other biochemical functions. It has been postulated that a genetic abnormality in metabolism may lead to the pathogenesis of migraine and that adding riboflavin may provide chemical precursors necessary to overcome this defect. To investigate this hypothesis, a study was performed in which migraineurs received high doses of riboflavin in a **placebo-controlled** trial. The results were promising: Migraineurs taking 400 mg of riboflavin for at least one month began experiencing fewer attacks, and this effect reached its maximum after three months. Riboflavin does not improve headache severity, duration, or associated symptoms, but it also has very few side effects. It discolors the urine and stool, turning them a bright orange or yellow. While the usual daily requirement of riboflavin is only 1.7 mg for men and 1.3 mg for women, the 400-mg dose recommended for migraine is not felt to be dangerous, as any unnecessary riboflavin passes out of the body through the urine.

Coenzyme Q10 is gaining some popularity among migraineurs as a possible prophylactic treatment. Coenzyme Q10 is a substance necessary in the production of energy by mitochondria. **Mitochondria** are located within cells and are where energy production takes place. They have also been implicated in the pathogenesis of migraine. Research suggests that when a person ingests coenzyme Q10, the functioning of the mitochondria are enhanced, which leads to fewer migraines. In at least two studies, coenzyme Q10 was shown to have a small beneficial effect after four weeks. Although it is safe,

Placebo-controlled

A comparison of a drug or treatment against an inert substance (**placebo**).

Mitochondria

The "powerhouses" of a cell; the energy-producing structures in cells.

this medication is expensive (costing as much as $50 per month as an out-of-pocket expense, because coenzyme Q10 is not covered by insurance). Much more research is needed to warrant widespread use of this product.

Other B vitamins—namely, B_6 and B_{12}—have also been suggested as potential migraine treatments. Vitamin B_{12} has been postulated to be helpful in migraine owing to its work as a nitric oxide scavenger. **Nitric oxide** has been implicated in the dilation of blood vessels. Dilation of the blood vessels occurs as a result of the activation of the neurotransmitter cascade described in Question 3, and it is believed to be responsible for stretching nerve endings, leading to the sensation of pain. With more vitamin B_{12} present to corral nitric oxide, it is believed that the vessels will be less reactive to this cascade.

Nitric oxide
A molecule that is involved in dilating blood vessels.

Vitamin B_6 is thought to be useful in treating so-called histamine headaches—that is, migraines precipitated by ingestion of wine and certain foods. This vitamin may be dangerous to the nervous system if taken in large quantities, however, so its use as a migraine therapy is generally not recommended. A better course of action is to avoid offending triggers.

Finally, vitamin A is occasionally mentioned as a possible agent for the treatment of headaches; however, there are no studies supporting its use. The lack of evidence mitigates against the use of vitamin A as a migraine therapy simply because of the potential danger to the brain and liver in the event of an overdose.

A mineral that is popular in the treatment of migraine is magnesium. While this substance is not a vitamin, it has been found to be depleted in many migraineurs. If given **intravenously** during an active attack, magnesium has

Intravenously
Administered by a catheter inserted into a vein.

been shown to be effective in relieving pain. However, this mode of administration may be cumbersome for some individuals. Many neurologists recommend that their migraine patients take 400 to 600 mg of magnesium daily, with the medication usually being found at local pharmacies and health food stores. To prevent migraines, it is best to take preparations with magnesium as the only ingredient. The most common side effects are diarrhea and stomach upset.

Several herbal supplements that do not require a prescription are used to treat migraines. Despite their over-the-counter status, these supplements may be quite effective and highly potent—but they may also interact with other medications you are taking and have undesirable side effects. In addition, they may not be as pure or as consistent in dose from pill to pill or from manufacturer to manufacturer as nonherbal medications. Because they are considered dietary supplements, these products' manufacture is not as tightly controlled as the manufacture of prescription medications. Before taking any herbal preparation, make sure you understand its intended use, dosing, side effects, and potential interactions with other medications. Always mention herbal remedies when you see a physician and take the bottle with you to your appointment. You may find these preparations extremely helpful in controlling your migraines if taken properly.

Always mention herbal remedies when you see a physician and take the bottle with you.

Feverfew (*Tanacetum parthenium*), also known as *bachelor's buttons*, is perhaps the most well known of the herbs for headache treatment. At the same time, it has perhaps the most checkered reputation. Feverfew has been implicated in the medication overuse (rebound) headaches described in Question 29. While scientists do not know exactly how this herb works to decrease migraine, the supplement is believed to act via the serotonin pathway. It has also been shown to affect **platelet aggregation**. Platelets are the cells that help with blood clotting, so this herbal supplement should be used with caution or not at all in patients taking aspirin, **warfarin**, **dipyridamole**, **tacrine**, and other drugs that affect the function of platelets. Finally, clinical trials studying the effectiveness of feverfew have produced mixed results. Many of my patients who tried this supplement did not find it to be helpful; many also find that its cost outweighs the additional benefit it brings to an ongoing regimen. Keep in mind, though, that these folks have severe enough headaches to seek the care of a physician. If your headaches are not that severe, you may find feverfew worth a try.

Petadolex® (*Petasites hybridus* extract), also known as *butterbur*, is another option. This herbal supplement is used as a prophylactic agent to decrease the number of headache episodes and to decrease the pain and duration of those episodes. It is believed to have anti-inflammatory effects and to play a role in the vascular phase of migraine. Petadolex® has been used for many years in Europe with success, and its use is increasing in the United States. The results of several well-designed studies lend credence to claims of its effectiveness in the treatment of migraine. Petadolex® is taken twice daily, with improvement generally being noted in one to three months. This herbal supplement is not known to interact with any of the commonly used abortive medications for migraine.

Other herbal remedies include menthol, peppermint, white willow bark tea, passionflower, and ginger. Many people use Tiger Balm®, a combination of menthol, camphor, eucalyptus, and lanolin that is rubbed across the neck or brow. Another patient of mine prefers white flower oil, a variant on Tiger Balm® that is easily found in most

---

TREATMENT AND THE DOCTOR'S VISIT

Platelet aggregation

The tendency of the clotting cells (platelets) to get together and form clots. These clots may lead to strokes in the brain.

Warfarin

A potent blood thinner used to prevent strokes and to prevent clots in heart patients. This medication also may put patients at risk for bleeding in the brain.

Dipyridamole

A medicine that is used to keep your platelets from clotting together. This medicine is used to help prevent strokes.

Tacrine

A medicine used to treat the symptoms of Alzheimer's disease.

Chinese shops. This stronger, more liquid form of Tiger Balm® also has a more pungent odor. I sometimes recommend peppermint oil or chewing peppermints, such as Altoids® or the sugar-free variety found in most grocery stores, as many anecdotal reports cite peppermint's soothing quality during a migraine. Interestingly, many of these botanicals have intense odors or flavors, which are often used to relieve nausea. Therefore, these alternatives may be particularly useful for those migraineurs who have a strong nausea component to their migraines. Although there are no controlled studies evaluating these oils, unguents, teas, and barks in the treatment or relief of migraine, they are unlikely to do you harm, and many patients report them to be soothing. In summary, these remedies should be considered as an adjunctive supportive measure to make you feel more comfortable as opposed to "treating" your migraine.

27. What type of side effects can I expect from medications?

Max's comment:

For years I used Advil® [ibuprofen] to treat my headaches. Then I developed hives and angioedema, which, when it occurred, was both frightening and disfiguring, since it affected my face, hands, and feet. While the hives were a daily occurrence, the angioedema would occur if I took an NSAID combined with any one of a number of foods that I am not allergic to under normal circumstances. It took a long time to realize that it was connected to taking Advil®. I have discontinued use of any NSAIDs, but that eliminates a large number of over-the-counter and prescription drugs. I have also taken Topamax® to prevent migraines but discontinued it due to a bad taste in my mouth, mood swings, and concern about the side effect of kidney stones. On the plus side, I had only 2 migraines in 6 months and lost 21 pounds.

The adverse effects of the drug overrode the positives, so I needed to seek other medications.

The side effects that people experience from the various medications prescribed for migraines vary from medication to medication and from person to person. In general, any new medication comes with side effects. The trick is to understand what to expect. The first step, before you leave the office with a new prescription, is to ask your physician what might be experienced after taking the medication. It sounds obvious, but after you have spent time going over your history and being examined, you may forget to ask questions. Sometimes these questions may interfere with your being able to take the medication when you buy it—if you buy it. Many of the prescriptions written are not filled, and those that are filled are never taken by the patient. Often just having medication available is reassuring to patients, so they do not take their pills. Therefore, be sure to ask any questions about the medication prescribed before you leave the office. Failing that, a good pharmacist will often be happy to answer any questions you might have.

Side effects of some of the more common medications are listed here. These side effects do not occur in all people, however, and many occur in only a small percentage of those taking the medicine.

Over-the-Counter Medications Used to Treat Individual Episodes

Acetaminophen: very well tolerated in most people.

Aspirin: gastrointestinal irritation and/or bleeding. Enteric-coated varieties may lessen these effects.

Nonsteroidal anti-inflammatory drugs (NSAIDs): gastrointestinal irritation and/or bleeding. Taking these medications with meals or crackers may lessen these effects.

Acetaminophen

A mild analgesic used to abort migraine attacks. It can be purchased over the counter.

Prescription Medications Used to Treat Individual Episodes

Butalbital (always used in combination with acetaminophen or aspirin and usually caffeine, although there are preparations without caffeine on the market): drowsiness (which may be offset if the preparation contains caffeine) and/or rash. Do not use this medication if you have an allergy to barbiturates. Also, watch for habituation and tolerance.

Ergotamine preparations: diarrhea, muscle cramps, nausea, tingling in the extremities.

Triptans: "weird" sensations such as warmth and pressure in the throat and upper chest or other parts of the body; tingling in extremities; sleepiness, dizziness, and nausea. A bad taste may be experienced with nasal preparations, and injection site reactions may be experienced with subcutaneous injections.

Prescription Medications Used to Prevent Episodes

Anticonvulsant Medications

Divalproex sodium: drowsiness, hair loss, tremor, weight gain, nausea.

Gabapentin: dizziness, unsteadiness, lethargy, swelling, weight gain.

Topiramate: fatigue, dizziness, unsteadiness, tingling in the fingers, nervousness, word-finding difficulties, weight loss, kidney stones. You must drink eight 10-ounce glasses of water per day while on this medicine. Increased intraocular pressure (glaucoma), "unmasking" of depression, or worsening of depression may also be seen.

Antidepressant Medications

Amitriptyline: drowsiness, dry mouth, weight gain, urinary retention, dizziness, rhythm problems with the heart. A related medication, nortriptyline, is often used by many physicians because, although it has similar side effects, they are generally less severe.

Selective serotonin reuptake inhibitors (SSRIs): drowsiness, nervousness, tremor, sexual dysfunction, insomnia, headache.

Phenelzine: gastrointestinal discomfort, malaise, tremors, dizziness on standing up.

Blood Pressure Medications

Beta blockers: slow heartbeat, depression, tiredness, sexual dysfunction, memory problems, worsening asthma, difficulty appreciating symptoms of hypoglycemia in diabetes.

Calcium-channel Blockers (depending on the medication): swelling of the ankles, dizziness, and nausea.

28. Are the medications for migraine addicting?

People frequently ask if they could become addicted to the medicines that their doctors prescribe. This book discusses many types of medicines. Of all of these medications, the narcotic analgesics are the only medicines that are truly potentially addicting if used incorrectly.

Narcotics are medications that contain an opioid, a substance that is used throughout health care for the treatment of moderate to severe pain. Opioids can take either natural or synthetic forms and have been used by humans in various settings for thousands of years. As recently as the early 1900s, opioids were available as over-the-counter drugs in the United States. To understand how narcotics are addicting, it is first important to understand the definition of addiction.

Unfortunately, the term "addiction" is often used incorrectly and many people, including healthcare professionals, often use the term loosely, sometimes confusing the meaning of the word. While taking narcotics may lead to addiction, this is only one of three possible outcomes seen with narcotics. These three separate forms are physical dependence, addiction, and tolerance.

Physical Dependence

Physical dependence is an *expected* and *normal* consequence that occurs as a reaction to taking certain medications, including narcotics. It is associated with withdrawal symptoms when the drug is stopped abruptly or when the dose is lowered too quickly. Physical dependence is a *common* effect that occurs in people who take opioid medications. It is expected and can be addressed by your physician.

Physical dependence differs from addiction. Undergoing physical changes when a drug is stopped qualifies as physical dependence, but it is not necessarily a sign of addiction. Typical withdrawal symptoms include sweating, chills, body aches, and flu-like symptoms. While these effects are not necessarily dangerous, they are unpleasant and should be discussed with your doctor.

Addiction

Addiction is a chronic disease that is associated with specific psychological and behavioral factors. Typically, addiction to opioids occurs in people who have a history of addiction or other psychiatric disorders such as depression or anxiety. Addiction may be defined as a compulsive, repeated use of a substance despite negative and harmful consequences. This state has been sometimes referred to as psychological dependence, although evidence now suggests that this disorder has genetic, neurobiological, and psychological components. Addiction is relatively rare when opioids are used properly and when there is no history of addiction in the patient or the patient's family. The overwhelming majority of patients who use opioid medications for pain relief do not develop addiction, though they can develop physical dependence.

If addiction does occur or you think pain medications are interfering with your ability to perform adequately in your work and interpersonal roles, speak to your physician immediately. While addiction is not common in pain patients who are monitored by a physician, it can occur and is a serious problem. If you have a history of addiction or have experienced problems with alcohol or any drugs, share this information with your doctor prior to starting any narcotic medication. A history of addiction does not exclude you from being treated with these medications, but your treatment should be under the direct guidance of your healthcare team.

Tolerance

Tolerance is a state of adaptation to a drug in which you might require more of the drug to receive the same desired effect. Your doctor will speak to you about this possibility if you find the medication is no longer having the same results. As with physical dependence, tolerance is a normal consequence of opioid painkillers and is not the same as addiction.

In the treatment of severe headaches, narcotics do have a place when they are administered under careful supervision. Some patients find these drugs to be very effective rescue medications when nothing else is working and will keep several doses in the house at all times. Likewise, some emergency room physicians use narcotics for intractable migraine when all else fails. There is also a nasal preparation (butorphanol [Stadol®]) that some patients find effective for severe headaches.

Perhaps the biggest drawback, however, are the side effects. Narcotics are sedating and constipating, and they can cause itching, unsteadiness, and *headache*. Codeine is a particular offender in this respect. This is not unusual: Many medications cause the same symptoms that they treat. In this case, because so many good alternatives are readily available, and because opioids have so many other negative side effects, more and more physicians are moving away from narcotics, except in very specialized circumstances under very close supervision.

If your doctor does prescribe narcotics, you can expect to sign a contract related to this use. Unfortunately, because of the substance abuse problem in our society, narcotics are tightly controlled, and their use and abuse among patients have prompted many doctors to lay out ground rules for refills, lost prescriptions, and other parameters; patients must agree to these ground rules prior to receiving controlled substances. Generally, these contracts protect everyone. If you and your physician decide that a narcotic controlled substance is an appropriate therapy for you and you are asked to sign a patient contract, do not feel offended. It is a common practice, and you are not being singled out.

29. I have come across the terms "rebound" and "medication overuse" headache. Are these just other names for addiction?

In the treatment of migraine, many patients find a medication that works very well for them. There is then a tendency to use this medication early in a headache episode to abort the headache. Patients are, in fact, encouraged to do so, and this practice makes physiological sense now that we have a better understanding of the neurobiology of migraine and the chemical cascades that occur as a migraine develops (see Question 3). One potential problem, however, is that patients may overuse the medicine. This overuse may then lead to the troubling phenomenon known as medication overuse headache.

Medication overuse headache is a well-recognized phenomenon that occurs when an abortive medication for headaches is taken on a daily basis. If a dose is missed, then a headache may develop. This, in turn, leads to taking medication again, except that now you need more of it to control the pain. Eventually more and more medication may be necessary to control the pain, but it may just be the absence of regular dosing of the medicine that leads to the pain.

You should work closely with your physician if you are on daily abortive medications (such as acetaminophen and aspirin) to assure that you are not overusing the medicine. Often you will be able to tell if this is occurring because you will notice that as soon as you miss a dose of medicine, the headache returns, as opposed to needing the medicine only intermittently. Using a calendar to monitor the pattern of your medicine usage every now and again is a useful way to guard against this possibility (see Question 53). On occasion, medication overuse headaches may be severe enough to drive patients to the emergency room seeking relief.

30. What if I am taking migraine medication and then find out I am pregnant? Will the medication harm my unborn child?

One of the most frustrating experiences of being pregnant is that once you are aware that you are pregnant, you are told to take no medications other than acetaminophen. The exceptions are medicines prescribed by your physician for chronic medical conditions that must be treated for you and your unborn child to remain safe. Your obstetrician may change you from one medicine to another one that treats the same disease and has potentially less harmful effects on a fetus; however, most physicians try to put those patients who are in their childbearing years on medications that are safe should the patient become pregnant.

Once told of this restriction, many women have a myriad of feelings regarding medications they took during the early weeks of pregnancy. These feelings may include guilt, fear, anger, or resignation, to name a few. These feelings may not be limited to prescription drugs, but may also extend to alcohol, tobacco, and recreational drugs. In general, medicines taken during the first two to three weeks of pregnancy (typically defined as the time since your last menstrual period) will either cause the fetus to spontaneously abort or will have no significant impact on the pregnancy and its outcome. It is imperative, however, that you discuss any and all medications that you take during this time with your obstetrician, including both prescribed and over-the-counter drugs.

During weeks 3 through 10 of a pregnancy, when the organs of the fetus are beginning to form, medications begin to affect organ formation. Medications that have such effects are classified by the Federal Drug Administration (FDA) based on what is known about them. After week 10, problems are usually related to damage to already formed organs and developing systems as well as to poor growth.

The biggest concern related to medication use in pregnancy is in the first trimester, when the major formation of organs occurs. Another time of concern is late in pregnancy, when medications may affect the changes that occur in the fetus at delivery. Always check with your physician if you have taken medications during the early weeks of your pregnancy and are concerned about the effects they may have had on your unborn fetus. Easily accessed national registries can provide information on certain medications and their effects during pregnancy.

In the United States, the FDA classifies all drugs according to their risk to the fetus (**Table 2**). Physicians use this classification in working with patients to come up with the best regimen for both the patient and her unborn child. Most, if not all, drugs given to the mother are essentially being given to the fetus simultaneously. As a consequence, the physician and patient must work together to decide on the best regimen. This regimen must take into consideration the risk to the fetus posed by the drug and the risk to the mother posed by a severe migraine. Migraines during pregnancy can lead to protracted vomiting, fluid losses, and lethargy, and these types of symptoms may in turn put the mother at risk for other medical complications.

Table 2 FDA classification of drugs.

Category	Description
A	Adequate, well-controlled studies in pregnant women have not shown an increased risk of fetal abnormalities.
B	Animal studies have revealed no evidence of harm to the fetus; however, there are no adequate and well-controlled studies in pregnant women. *or* Animal studies have shown an adverse effect, but adequate and well-controlled studies in pregnant women have failed to demonstrate a risk to the fetus.
C	Animal studies have shown an adverse effect, and there are no adequate and well-controlled studies in pregnant women. *or* No animal studies have been conducted, and there are no adequate and well-controlled studies in pregnant women.
D	Studies—adequate, well-controlled, or observational—in pregnant women have demonstrated a risk to the fetus. However, the benefits of therapy may outweigh the potential risk.
X	Studies—adequate, well-controlled, or observational—in animals or pregnant women have demonstrated positive evidence of fetal abnormalities. The use of the product is contraindicated in women who are or may become pregnant.

In the FDA classification system, Category A drugs pose no risk to a fetus, but very few drugs fall into this category. Category X drugs are contraindicated in pregnancy, meaning that probably no physician will prescribe them. Drugs in Categories B, C, and D may be discussed by you and your physician, and may be prescribed under certain circumstances with a full understanding of the risks and benefits to you and your unborn child. You also may be asked to sign a form outlining these risks and benefits, acknowledging that you understand them. Because of the relative unknowns in prescribing medications during pregnancy and our society's concern regarding harm to the unborn child, it is likely that you will be encouraged to use nonmedicinal approaches to migraine such as those outlined in Questions 89 to 99.

In migraine treatment during pregnancy, acetaminophen is recommended in combination with nonmedication approaches, such as relaxation techniques, meditation, biofeedback, acupuncture, and exercise, to name a few. Should you need more medication for acute treatment of migraine, other options are available but must be discussed with your neurologist. Medications that your neurologist will probably not prescribe during your pregnancy include the triptans or any preparations containing ergotamines. Other medications that probably will not be recommended during pregnancy are the preventive medicines. These medicines tend to be those with higher risks and may be less necessary, as many women experience fewer headaches as their pregnancy progresses. However, if your migraines become so troubling that they pose more risk to you than the medications themselves, your neurologist and obstetrician will work together to come up with the best regimen to meet your needs. Medications that have been used in pregnancy with some success include the beta blockers and tricyclic antidepressants. Nonpharmacological approaches are also very important, as are monitoring and decreasing migraine triggers. Any vitamins and herbs should be taken under a physician's supervision during pregnancy, as many of these supplements can cause bleeding or other symptoms that may prove dangerous in pregnancy.

Maintaining an awareness of the risks of any medication you are taking prior to becoming pregnant is especially important. Discuss these risks with your physician. If you miss a period, you should contact your physician about immediately stopping any medication that has a high risk until you know if you are pregnant. And of course, good healthcare practices fall into this category as well. Smoking and recreational drugs have health implications for both you and your unborn child. Therefore, working on stopping these habits before you become pregnant puts you way ahead of the game. Alcohol is a migraine trigger for many women; if you have not cut back on your intake for this reason, doing so in preparation for a baby is another good reason. More information can be found on the website *http://www.hon.ch/Dossier/MotherChild/preg_drugs/index.html#source1*, and in the Appendix.

31. Is it safe to take my migraine medications while I am breastfeeding?

Medications pass through breast milk to an infant to varying degrees depending on the medicine. In general, a breastfeeding infant ingests a very small proportion of the medication taken by the mother. Although many medications may be detectable in breast milk, they are not necessarily harmful to an infant. Nevertheless, their risks and benefits should always be discussed with your physician.

Other strategies for treating migraines may also be helpful while breastfeeding, such as adjusting doses around your nursing schedule and treating just acute episodes as opposed to using preventive medication plus acute treatment. Your physician may also switch you to medications that are known to be safer in breastfeeding until your baby is no longer nursing. The safest course of action is to speak to your neurologist and pediatrician about the specific medication that you are taking. Make sure you clearly understand all the risks and benefits of the medication and the alternatives available to you. You should also ask your pediatrician about any signs to watch for in your infant that should be brought to the pediatrician's attention.

32. I've heard a lot about Botox® for headaches. How does it work to prevent migraines?

New medications and treatments are being developed and used on huge numbers of people every day for any number of diseases. Because migraine is so common, it does not take long for sufferers to notice that a medicine or treatment for one disease may also help their headaches. It is not unusual for a patient to report this information to his or her physician, who then tells a colleague, who subsequently notices the same effect in his or her patients, and so on. Before long, studies are designed to test the new treatment. In addition, physicians often use these medicines with patients who have failed other treatments and are miserable with their pain. Botox® is one such medication.

Botulinum toxin (Botox®) is produced by the bacteria *Clostridium botulinum.* When injected into muscle, the toxin interrupts the transmission of chemicals in the muscle needed to allow the muscle to contract. As a result, the muscle becomes paralyzed. This effect lasts for only the short term, however: Reversal begins in three months and is usually complete in six months. When Botox® is injected into the face, it leads to a loss of wrinkles as well as some change in facial expression. Other side effects are the development of antibodies to the toxin that render it less effective (less than 1%) or that produce drooping eyelids and scarring at the injection site. Finally, patients receiving injections for wrinkles and painful muscle spasms have noticed an interesting side effect of decreased headache. It has been postulated that Botox® reduces the activation of trigeminal nerve fibers and neurons in the brain stem, making it more difficult to trigger a migraine.

Botulinum toxin (Botox®)

A toxin produced by a bacterium that causes paralysis of muscles. This toxin may prevent migraines when injected into muscles of the face and neck.

When clinicians began using Botox® to remove wrinkles, they found that many of their patients' migraines became less troublesome following the injections. Neurologists have begun doing trials to further explore the benefits of Botox®. Some trials have shown that the toxin is an effective treatment for headaches, whereas others do not support its use for migraine. Although not approved by the FDA for use in migraine treatment, many neurologists are using Botox® in their patients with varying degrees of success. Generally, it is reserved for patients who have severe migraine and who have failed other treatments. Early trials have found that as many as 50% of patients find relief; however, more studies are needed.

Botox® is certainly an option for patients who are willing to try newer treatment options and who can afford the expense. It is quite expensive and is not generally covered by insurance for migraine treatment. It is recommended that if you are interested in Botox® for your migraines that you consider the following questions:

- Are you currently dissatisfied enough with your current migraine regimen that you feel it could be improved?
- Are you willing to try a new treatment that involves needles and injections in your face?
- Are you able to afford a treatment such as Botox®, or could you budget your finances to fit it in every three months?

If you have answered yes to these questions, Botox® may be an option for you.

33. It sounds as though Botox® might have more downsides than benefits. Why should I even consider it?

Botox® is a preventive treatment. Most neurologists will consider you for preventive treatment when you experience one migraine per week, or when your migraines are interfering with home life and/or causing absenteeism from work, or when you are taking so many medications on an as-needed basis that it is felt to be better, cheaper, and/or safer to have fewer migraines. Many preventive treatments are quite costly, must be taken one to three times daily, and may have unpleasant side effects or may not work. Consider, then, Botox®, which involves a visit to the doctor every three months for injections.

If Botox® works for you and you can afford it, it may well be an option as a preventive treatment. While paying for Botox® requires out-of-pocket expenditures (i.e., it is not covered by most insurance for the treatment of migraine), and the cost is in the $300 to $1500 range for one treatment, this medication may well be worth the expense if you add up the deductibles for other medications incurred over a three-month period.

When you are choosing a neurologist to deliver Botox® injections, be sure that the physician has experience in the technique, and that he or she takes the time to explain the procedure as well as all of the risks and benefits to you. Also, ask whether the physician is participating in any clinical trials involving Botox®. If so, you may be able to join the study if you meet its inclusion criteria. This is a great way to defray the cost of the Botox® and see if the treatment works. Read Question 46 on clinical trials before agreeing to participate in a clinical trial.

34. How long will I have to take medication(s) to control my migraines?

Not surprisingly, everyone is different when it comes to answering this question. The answer will depend on how old you are when you start experiencing headaches, how severe and how often your headaches occur, and how much they interfere with your lifestyle. It also may depend on your personal preference and style about taking medications. One of the most interesting things I have noticed in my practice is that my migraine patients are the most hesitant to take medications of any sort. I am not sure if this reluctance is related to having migraines per se, but over the years I have treated many different neurological disorders requiring daily or "as needed" medication. Many of these diseases are not as disabling or as painful as migraine, yet my migraine patients are the most fearful of becoming addicted or dependent on medicines. Or, they simply do not like to take pills of any sort. While I strongly encourage all of my patients to make use of alternative approaches, vitamins and supplements, and lifestyle changes, chances are that medications will still be needed if their migraines are severe enough to seek medical attention.

If you are given only abortive medications such as triptans, you may need to take these medicines until your migraines fade with menopause, if you are a woman, or decrease in severity and frequency, if you are a man. If you are taking a prophylactic medication and you have a very good response, many physicians may try to taper you off after six months of good control to see if you can get by with only abortive treatment. For many people, prophylaxis may improve their migraine control, but may be needed for a longer term. On occasion, patients who are doing well on medications may get worse in their control despite their best efforts to control triggers and otherwise modify their lifestyle. For these patients, I may recommend that they taper all prophylactic medications for a drug holiday and either restart the same medication or try another agent.

We now view migraine as a chronic disease with episodic attacks. It begins in young adulthood and peaks in middle age. If you consider this model, there is every likelihood that eventually you will be able to throw away your prescription pill bottles and get by with the occasional over-the-counter preparation.

35. When should I see a doctor for my migraines?

Migraines vary in terms of how severe they are and how frequently they occur. Many times migraines are relieved by rest and relaxation or by over-the-counter medications in low doses, such as acetaminophen or aspirin. Some people get the best relief from ibuprofen. While headaches might occur quite frequently, the fact that they go away with over-the-counter medicines or rest often keeps many individuals from seeing a physician. Many people may mention their headaches to their primary care physician or gynecologist during a routine visit, but if they are relieved by over-the-counter medications, often the physician will make a note of their presence and recommend a continuation of the use of these medications.

Some people find that their headaches change over time, with new symptoms accompanying them or an increase in severity and/or frequency. Mild headaches may change in character over time. Dull headaches may become more intense and throbbing. Headaches that crescendo over the course of a day with the maximal discomfort occurring at night may become headaches that wake the person up and reach their maximal and intense pain in a short period of time. These kinds of changes may signal the onset of migraine in a person with tension headaches. These new headaches may often be treated with larger doses of over-the-counter medications and sleeping in a dark, quiet room. If the migrainous headache is not so easily treated, this may be the time to see a primary care physician or even a neurologist. These changes also may signal the onset of other neurological disorders that warrant medical evaluation.

Gastric reflux

The regurgitation of stomach acids into the esophagus (the tube-like organ connecting the throat to the stomach). Medications and certain foods may cause this problem to occur.

The best time to see a doctor for your migraines is when you feel that you can no longer manage them on your own for whatever reason.

Many patients use over-the-counter medications with good success but notice that over time they gradually become less effective. These individuals may find themselves increasing the dose in a way that is alarming or find that what worked previously is just not doing the trick. Or they may have a medical problem, such as **gastric reflux**, that prohibits the use of certain over-the-counter preparations. Patients with stomach problems and gastric reflux or peptic ulcers may not be able to easily use a nonsteroidal anti-inflammatory drug (NSAID) such as aspirin, ibuprofen, or naproxyn sodium, for example. If acetaminophen is not effective and NSAIDs are contraindicated, prescription medications may be necessary to relieve the headache.

In summary, the best time to see a doctor for your migraines is when you can no longer manage them on your own for whatever reason. This reason may be medical, psychological, or neurological. Or perhaps you simply need more information and reassurance. Any of these are good reasons for consulting a physician, and you should feel comfortable seeking medical care for your migraines.

Max's comment:

It took me a long time to acknowledge that I was having migraines. I think I had a lot of denial about having them. I had always had headaches, with some lasting up to 36 hours in spite of taking over-the-counter treatments, but I continued to believe that they were "normal" headaches. It was only recently (within the last two years) that I described my headaches to my physician accurately, and he has prescribed medications that are specific to migraine treatment. Because I have a trusting, ongoing relationship with my neurologist (because of a seizure disorder), it was relatively easy for me to discuss my symptoms with him and address the issue. This did not occur until I was in my late fifties.

36. What kind of doctor should I see for my migraines?

Cherie's comment:

After speaking to many migraineurs and seeking a cure for my headaches, I have found that most doctors do not know how to treat headaches. The diagnosis of a migraine is often overlooked or not treated with the importance it deserves. Someone who suffers with headaches on a regular basis needs to be reassured that a physician is taking their symptoms seriously. Migraines are not always a symptom of another illness; they are a serious and debilitating condition unto itself. I believe that in most cases only a neurologist is qualified to meet this task, and that neurologist has to be the right match for you. I have been blessed with mine because she is there for me when I need her, and her goal is to keep me as pain free as possible.

Primary care physicians or gynecologists are usually the first type of doctor many patients see for their migraines. Generally, the person complains of headaches to this physician during a regular visit for another medical problem. These doctors can often initiate the first line of treatment for all headache types and make a diagnosis. They may also provide reassurance that the headache is not dangerous. They may perform a general physical examination and blood work to rule out possible medical causes for headache and review all medications that you may be taking to assure that you are not taking a medication that may be causing your headache.

Your primary care physician may refer you to a neurologist if you do not respond to the medications he or she prescribes or if there is a concern about the type of headaches you are experiencing. Alternatively, they may make this kind of referral because they want a second opinion and/or to reassure you. You also may go directly to a neurologist for your migraine. General neurologists consider the diagnosis and management of migraine an essential part of their practice. In fact, headache is one of the most common disorders that neurologists evaluate and treat.

37. What is a neurologist?

Many people confuse neurologists and neurosurgeons. While both types of physicians deal with the nervous system, the neurologist does not perform surgery. Neurologists take care of diseases of the brain, nerves, and muscles. These disorders include headache, stroke, epilepsy, Parkinson's disease, multiple sclerosis, Alzheimer's disease, and muscular dystrophy, to name a few. Neurologists also take care of some rare diseases that you may have heard of, such as **Lou Gehrig's disease (amyotrophic lateral sclerosis), Guillain-Barré syndrome**, and the disease that inspired the movie *Lorenzo's Oil* (adrenoleukodystrophy). They also see patients with dizziness and back pain as well as tumors of the nervous system. A neurologist usually sees patients on referral from other physicians,

Lou Gehrig's disease (amyotrophic lateral sclerosis)
The disease that struck down the baseball player Lou Gehrig. This disease causes a weakness in the muscles of the limbs and throat, rendering patients unable to move, speak, and breathe on their own.

Guillain-Barré syndrome
A neurological disease in which a person becomes weak in a gradually ascending pattern. It may affect breathing as well.

Lorenzo's Oil
A movie about a rare neurological disease that afflicts children. This movie illustrates the role that neurologists play in caring for patients with rare and devastating neurological diseases.

but often patients seek care from neurologists directly. Neurologists initially may see a patient in consultation and then continue seeing the patient in follow-up visits if warranted by the patient's neurological problem.

Neurologists are specially trained in identifying and treating neurological diseases and in the art of performing the neurological examination. The complete neurological examination is an in-depth examination of the brain, nerves, and muscles, and an assessment of cognitive function and memory. Neurologists prescribe many types of medications and perform many procedures to assess muscle and nerve functions, such as **electromyography (EMG)**, brain wave tests, and **electroencephalography (EEG)**, and they inject substances into muscles such as botulinum toxin. These physicians may work in hospitals, clinics, private offices, and medical schools. They work closely with neurosurgeons, taking care of patients together to assure the best possible outcome for patients who need surgery.

Many neurologists are currently performing important research in genetics and on the diseases that afflict our population, to better understand them and to develop new treatments and methods of prevention. Some examples include stroke, epilepsy, and migraine. Neurology is a small, but important specialty—as many as one-half to two-thirds of all hospitalized patients suffer from one or more neurological problems.

Finally, many neurologists make their living solely in the area of headache and migraine. These physicians see primarily patients with headache, do research in headache and migraine, and manage the headache centers where patients go for premiere headache treatment. They also teach other neurologists about migraine and

Electromyography (EMG)

A test performed by a neurologist to assess muscle and nerve function. Fine-gauge needles are gently inserted into muscles to measure their electrical activity.

Electroencephalography (EEG)

A test performed by neurologists to assess brain waves. It is performed by applying electrodes to the scalp to measure the electrical activity of the brain for 20 minutes or longer.

headache. This responsibility is especially important because this is a rapidly evolving field, and headache is a disorder that affects such a large portion of our society.

38. When should I see a neurologist for my headaches?

Approximately 2% of migraineurs see a neurologist for their treatment. When primary care physicians refer their patients, they generally have a good reason for doing so. Either they believe that they have exhausted their armamentarium of treatment, or they may be unsure of the diagnosis. Often patients go straight to a neurologist if they are not happy with the current management of their headaches.

Neurologists treat simple, straightforward migraines as well as more complicated, refractory migraines. A neurologist will do a complete neurological examination and be able to discuss your concerns and fears about the possibility of a diagnosis other than migraine. Such a physician also will decide whether a brain scan is needed. Finally, a neurologist will be able to design the most up-to-date treatment plan with you, taking into consideration the most recent research, available medications, and your lifestyle.

You also may be referred to a headache center. These centers are run by the top neurologists in the country specializing in headache and migraine. Headache centers are multidisciplinary, in that they offer medical, nursing, psychological, psychiatric, and psychosocial support to the headache patient. They often offer inpatient options for the patient with refractory headaches and usually participate in many clinical trials involving the latest treatment approaches.

One thing is certain: If you are already seeing a physician and receiving medication for your headaches, and you decide to see a neurologist, it is imperative that you tell your physician that you would like to see a neurologist. Your physician may give you a referral or you may use the National Headache Foundation (*http://www.headaches.org*) and the American Council for Headache Education (*http://www.achenet.org*) to obtain the names of physicians specializing in the treatment of headache in your area.

39. What is a pain specialist?

You may be referred to a pain specialist if your migraines are complicated by other pain syndromes that could benefit from the therapies offered by the pain specialist. Pain specialists are often anesthesiologists, but they may be neurologists or psychiatrists. They tend to work in pain management centers, which are similar to headache centers in many ways. For example, pain centers are multidisciplinary in nature, offering medical, nursing, psychological, psychiatric, and psychosocial support. The main difference is that pain centers focus on many different types of pain rather than only headache. Such centers may be located in hospitals, in clinics, and in private settings.

Physicians working in pain centers often perform invasive procedures, such as anesthetic blocks in the spinal area and **trigger point** injections in muscles and tissues. These injections are often helpful in alleviating pain that occurs secondary to migraines in the neck muscles or pain that may precipitate migraines.

Trigger point

A spot in a muscle where if touched can elicit pain or radiation of pain. If injected with a steroid or anesthetic this pain is relieved.

Other physicians who may specialize in headache include internists, family physicians, and dentists.

Psychiatrist

A medical doctor who specializes in treating mental, emotional, and behavioral disorders such as depression and anxiety. Psychiatrists are physicians and thereby can prescribe medication to treat a wide variety of mental health problems.

Whether you choose a neurologist, anesthesiologist, or **psychiatrist** for your headache care, you should make sure that the physician has an interest and/or expertise in patients with headache. While this may sound obvious, sometimes people are referred to physicians who are "great"—but unfortunately in another specialty area.

40. When I see a physician for my migraines, what kind of examination will the doctor perform?

Often the history is the most useful aspect of the doctor's visit, as he or she attempts to understand and classify your headache type. A physician will spend lots of time asking you questions about your headaches (e.g., how long they last, how severe they are, what makes them worse, and what makes them better). This interview will allow for a better assessment of the type of pain you are having. It is also helpful if you write down your symptoms prior to your visit to the doctor. The doctor will want to know which types of symptoms you have and when they occur during your headache. If you plan to see a physician for your headaches, it will be very useful for you to keep a log of the symptoms that accompany your headache (either during or after, depending on how sick you feel). The doctor may also want to know when you experience your headaches and if they are related to particular events or triggers. If you are a woman, do they occur prior to your periods? Do they occur when you are stressed? Do they occur once a week or once every six months? A diary and headache questionnaire are provided in the Appendix to help you prepare for your visit.

The next step is a general physical exam, if you have not recently had one. This exam is typically performed by your primary care physician. The first thing to expect is an evaluation of your vital signs—specifically, your blood pressure, pulse, temperature, and rate of breathing. More recently, a fifth vital sign was added to the classic foursome: the evaluation of pain. Usually a physician will ask you to rate your pain on a scale of 0 to 10 using a mark along a line such as the one below (**Figure 3**).

Another method of assessing pain severity relies on a series of facial cartoons exhibiting increasing amounts of pain in their expressions (**Figure 4**). This scale may be especially helpful with children.

Next, the physician will perform a routine physical exam. As part of this exam, he or she will listen to your heart, lungs, and the large vessels in your neck, and examine your abdomen.

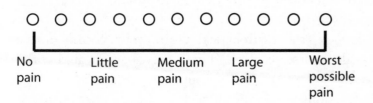

No pain   Little pain   Medium pain   Large pain   Worst possible pain

Figure 3 Typical pain scale.

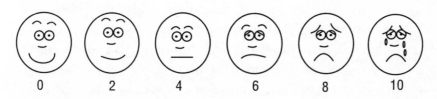

0   2   4   6   8   10

Figure 4 Cartoon pain scale.

Many maneuvers will be done to test your neurological system. The neurological examination is generally normal in the patient with migraine, but it must be done to assure there are no other causes of the migraine that might inspire concern. Some of these problems may cause focal neurological deficits—that is, patterns of numbness or weakness that may signify an underlying disorder or lesion.

Many internists or primary care physicians will perform a neurological exam, whereas others will refer you to a neurologist for a more detailed examination. The neurological examination is taught to all physicians in medical school; however, owing to its length and complexity, many primary care physicians rely on neurologists' expertise in performing the exam. Neurologists spend years of training to understand the nuances of the exam and its interpretation. In fact, neurology is one of the few specialties where the neurologist must examine a patient in the presence of other experienced neurologists to become certified by the American Board of Psychiatry and Neurology.

Cranial nerves

Nerves located in the head that control vision, facial expression, swallowing, hearing, eye movements, and sensation of the face and mouth.

Optic nerve

The cranial nerve that conveys vision. The end of this nerve is actually visible to physicians when they look into the eye.

During the neurological exam, your **cranial nerves** will be assessed first. These nerves are located within the skull and control the muscles, sensations, and other functions in your head, neck, and face. The neurologist will check your eye movements by having you look at his or her finger as it is moved from side to side; this tests the muscles of your eyes. Next, the doctor will shine a light into your eyes and into the back of your eyeball to check the functioning of your **optic nerve**, the nerve that mediates your vision. Next, the nerves that control the expression of your face; the movement of your tongue, neck, swallowing; and your hearing will be tested. You will be asked to stick out your tongue, show your teeth, and push your head sideways against the examiner's hand. To test your hearing, a tuning fork will be placed near your ear as well as on the bone behind your ear. Your gag reflex may be tested with a soft cotton swab dabbed against the back of your throat.

Your muscles will be tested for their strength, tone, and bulk. You may be asked to differentiate between sharp and dull objects placed against your skin as sensation is tested. Your elbows, knees, and ankles will be tapped with a reflex hammer, and a blunt object will be used to scratch the soles of your feet.

You may also be asked to perform some simple tests of coordination. These tests may consist of tapping your fingers and/or toes, touching your nose with your index finger, and walking in a straight line.

All of these tests are used to assist the physician in determining whether all of the portions of your **peripheral and central nervous systems** are functioning correctly. After they are complete, your doctor may ask you some questions to assess your memory. Often the neurologist can assess these functions through the interview process, but specific questions may be asked at the beginning or the end of the exam. If you feel that you are experiencing memory loss or are less sharp since the onset of your migraines, make sure that you mention this issue so that your memory may be evaluated more fully.

Peripheral and central nervous system

The nervous system is composed of a central portion that includes the brain and spinal cord, and a peripheral portion that includes the peripheral nerves, nerve endings, and muscles.

41. When do I need an x-ray for my migraines?

Plain skull x-rays were ordered more routinely in the past for headaches than they are today. With the advent of computerized axial tomography (CAT) scans and magnetic resonance imaging (MRI), both of which reveal brain structures in much greater detail, plain x-rays are now rarely used in the diagnostic work-up of headaches. The exception might be in case of trauma, where skull x-rays have some value in demonstrating fractures. To inspect the brain itself and any pathology that may be present, however, these images have limited value. As you can see from the skull film below (**Figure 5**), not much can be said about the brain from this picture!

X-rays of the upper peripheral and central nervous systems (neck bones) may be valuable in assessing for fractures and alignment of bones. In general, however, their use in the diagnostic work-up of headache is limited, as MRI is used to evaluate the **cervical spine** as well. For all these reasons, you are unlikely to have a standard x-ray done as part of a routine evaluation of your headache. If imaging is warranted, a CAT scan or MRI is more likely to be performed.

Cervical spine

The upper portion of the spine or neck. The spinal cord in this portion of the spine sends nerves to the arms and the back of the head.

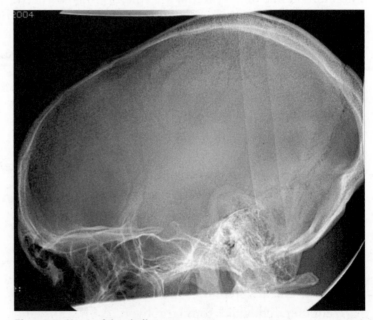

Figure 5 X-ray of the skull.

42. Should my doctor be ordering an MRI or CAT scan for headaches?

An MRI or CAT scan is needed only if your physician is worried about something other than a migraine. Many physicians will not order a brain scan if the patient's history is consistent with migraine and the neurological examination is normal.

This approach may be frustrating to the migraineur. Too often migraine sufferers feel as though they need to have some physical evidence of an illness to justify all their pain and disability. Migraine is a significant and disabling illness, and a normal neurological examination may prove frustrating as opposed to reassuring. Friends and family members may encourage the sufferer to "doctor shop" to "find out what is really wrong" when there is dissatisfaction with a diagnosis based on no abnormal physical findings on examination. This practice can lead to more stress and frustration, and put the migraine sufferer in the awkward position of not being perceived as adequately taking care of his or her own healthcare needs when, in fact, just the opposite is true. For this reason, many physicians will order an MRI or CAT scan for patients in whom they feel it will be reassuring.

A caveat is in order here: In any random scan of the "normal" population, lesions will be found. Because the area imaged is the brain, incidental findings unrelated to the headache may lead to great anxiety for the patient even though the lesion may be benign and of no consequence. Of course, in rare cases an incidental finding proves fortuitous and life-saving. Because none of these outcomes can be predicted with any good reliability for a specific individual, it is imperative that you discuss all possible findings, outcomes, and ramifications of brain scanning. If you are someone who cannot possibly go one more day without knowing that you absolutely do not have a brain tumor despite all medical reassurances, then a brain scan may be indicated. If you are someone who would worry incessantly if a benign abnormality were found in your brain despite medical assurances that it would never cause harm, then that possibility would need to be weighed as well. Another point to remember is that a scan on a given day is just that—it pictures your brain on that day but does not necessarily speak to the future.

If your physician decides to order a scan of your brain, the next decision is whether to order a CAT scan or MRI (**Figure 6**). Some types of headache are best evaluated with a CAT scan; others are best assessed with MRI. In some cases you may even have both types of imaging done. CAT scans can demonstrate the various structures in the brain as well as bone, blood, and some types of infections. MRI is more useful where fine

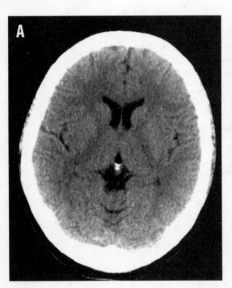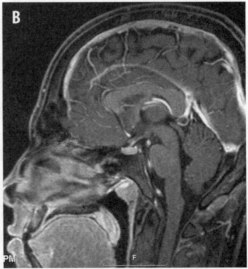

Figure 6 **(A)** Computerized axial tomography (CAT) scan **(B)** Magnetic resonance imaging (MRI)

details of normal brain structures or the delineation of lesions is needed. Both imaging techniques are often used in conjunction with contrast agents, which are injected into a blood vessel, usually in your arm. These agents enhance the various anatomical structures and lesions that are typically found in the brain and surrounding tissues.

You should always notify the radiologist prior to any study if you are pregnant, are nursing, or have any allergies, especially to iodine. If you are pregnant, there is no absolutely risk-free radiological study. If you must have a scan, discuss all of the risks and benefits to you and your fetus before you have the scan, and make sure you have all your questions answered to your satisfaction.

Once you have completed the scan, it is a good idea to ask the receptionist at the imaging center or radiologist's office when the films will be available to your physician. It is very frustrating to have a scan done, only to have to wait several more weeks for the results. Also, discuss with your physician how you will obtain the results of your scan. Make sure you know whether to call, come in for a visit, have the results faxed to you, pick up the films yourself, and so forth.

It is always recommended that you try not to interpret the films or the radiologist's report yourself. **"Medi-speak"** is often frightening to the layperson and is frequently misinterpreted. This misinterpretation can lead to more anxiety and stress—and even more headaches. If you pick up your films and an enclosed report, your first stop should be your physician's office, not the Internet!

Medi-speak

Tendency to speak using medical terms the listener may not understand.

43. I am claustrophobic. What if my physician orders an MRI?

Claustrophobic

Fear or extreme discomfort in a dark and/or enclosed space.

Many people are **claustrophobic**—that is, they fear small, closed-in spaces. An MRI machine is essentially a large tube-like structure, which allows very little space around you during the scan. For this reason, people who suffer from claustrophobia might find an MRI difficult to tolerate.

Several options are available in such case. One option is to find out whether an open MRI is accessible to you. These machines can provide high-quality pictures and are much less threatening to the claustrophobic individual.

Another option is to ask for administration of a mild prescription sedative during the scan. If this option is chosen, several things must be taken into consideration. First, you must be accompanied to the scan, and you may not drive yourself home. Second, you should ask your physician how quickly the sedative that you are given will work. All too often, the sedative is taken immediately before the scan, providing only minimal sedation during the scan but treating the individual to a quite relaxing post-scan period. Ask your physician about the type of medication used. Often people know in advance how they react to the various sedatives used in such cases. Most physicians use benzodiazepines, which is a class of drugs that includes Valium®, Librium®, Ativan®, and others. Let your physician know if you prefer one of these sedatives. It is better to take an agent with which you are familiar and comfortable than to combine the anxiety of taking a new medicine with the anxiety of undergoing the scan.

44. How will I know that the doctor is not missing something and making the wrong diagnosis?

Although there is no guarantee that a physician will always make a correct diagnosis, physicians are practiced in evaluating patients for specific diagnoses in their specialty. While we often think of medicine as a science, it is an art as well. When you go to a physician, he or she will request that you tell your story and will ask questions about your history and that of your family, your habits, and your social background. While listening and examining you, the physician is synthesizing all of this information and looking for patterns and/or themes that are consistent with certain diagnoses or groups of diseases. Often it seems as though you have barely finished telling your story when the physician is nodding his or her head and moving on to labeling your problem. Physicians become expert in recognizing the illnesses and problems that they see over and over again.

After completing medical school, physicians spend three to four years in residency learning to recognize these patterns, and to evaluate and manage the various diseases in their specialty, while being supervised by experienced physicians. Following residency, many go on to do an even more specialized fellowship in their field. Given this extensive training, the physician may be able to quickly recognize the pattern you describe while telling your story and begin to formulate a diagnosis.

Next, the doctor will want to obtain information more specific to the diagnosis being considered, refining the formulation. At this point, you may be asked more specific questions. It is important that you do not try to give "right" answers. Second-guessing what you think a physician might want to hear, trying to be a "good patient," and overstating your symptoms so the doctor will "believe" you and "understand" that you are in real pain are never good strategies. Simply tell your own truth.

Your physician gets only a glimpse into your life and headache story. Be sure it is a meaningful and candid one.

Keep in mind the physician has anywhere from 10 to 60 minutes to hear your story, understand your problem, and come up with a treatment plan. Essentially, your physician gets only a glimpse into your life and headache story. Be sure it is a meaningful and candid one.

45. I sometimes get tongue-tied at the doctor's office and leave not understanding what I was told or what I am to do. Is there any way to make my visits to my headache physician more productive?

Max's comment:

It's difficult for me to describe my symptoms or to remember everything that I want to tell my doctor. So, before going to my appointment, I like to review my problem list with my wife. We "rehearse" the list and, if necessary, I write [the issues] down and take the list with me. I am fortunate that I have been seeing the same neurologist for many years, and we have a positive relationship. He has been my doctor since I developed a seizure disorder, so we are well known to each other and he understands my communication style.

Everyone at one time has had the experience of going to the doctor's office and leaving frustrated, feeling that their questions weren't answered. You may be confused about the causes and treatment of your migraines and hope to get answers from the visit with your doctor. If this doesn't happen, you may feel discouraged or even irritated by the experience. This problem can be made worse if you aren't feeling well and are having a migraine at the time of the visit. Your memory may not be great that day, and you may have forgotten any questions you had. You are not alone in this experience.

It is important to establish a good relationship with your physician. When patients feel trusted and feel as if they are being listened to—*really listened to*—they feel better about their visit and will often do better in their treatment. The "right chemistry" is as important as the doctor's expertise.

When you go to the doctor for your migraines, make sure you are ready to answer the following questions, or at least make sure your headache history touches on these points. These items are a useful starting point for thinking about your migraines, and you may even find patterns emerging as you do so. Once you have started treatment, you will also be able to note the changes in the story as you gain more control over your migraines.

- When did your migraines start? How old were you? Do you remember your first one?
- How often do you have your migraines?
- How many different types of migraines do you have?
- Describe your typical migraine. If you have more than one type, be able to describe all types.
- How would you rate the severity of your pain?
- What are your headache triggers? (See Question 55 for more on triggers.)
- For women, are your migraines related to your periods? Are you menopausal or perimenopausal (three to five years before menopause, a time when estrogen levels begin to fall)?

- What makes your migraines better/worse?
- Do you take medications? Which ones? Do you have allergies to any medications?
- How often do your headache medicines work?
- What percentage of your headaches impair your ability to function?
- Is there a history of migraine in your family? In whom?
- Do you have any significant medical problems? Do you take medications for these problems?

While these questions are by no means exhaustive, if you have thought about them prior to seeing the physician, the history-taking portion of your visit will be much more productive.

To make the visit as productive as possible, it pays to plan in advance. Write your questions down before leaving home. Practice what you want to say. Put the most important questions at the top of the list. Be sure that you understand the answers. If you do not, ask the questions again or perhaps rephrase them until you are clear on the answer. You should also feel free to write down the things the doctor tells you. Don't rely on your memory. Often people are nervous in the doctor's office, and there are times your memory may not be the sharpest due to a headache episode.

When your visit is finishing and you and your physician are going over your treatment plan, you can take several steps to assure that you do not arrive home with many unanswered questions.

First, it is imperative that you understand the treatment plan and that this plan is one that you participate in developing. In other words, can you live with your

To make the visit as productive as possible, it pays to plan in advance.

treatment plan? If you are fearful of taking any type of medications and the doctor gives you three prescriptions, you should discuss your hesitations about taking medication. Perhaps alternatives exist, such as those discussed elsewhere in this book. Alternatively, this point may be a good juncture at which you and your physician discuss what your goals are and exactly how you will achieve them. It may be that a trial of one medication is a better starting point. This is just one example, but it highlights the importance of speaking up if you feel that the proposed treatment plan won't work for you. Usually physicians are happy to get your point of view and hear your concerns, and they will typically work with you in a way that will make you comfortable. The art of doctoring involves this type of relationship building, which is important in the development of a successful and trusting therapeutic relationship.

Next, be sure that you understand all instructions about your medications and their side effects. To do so, you need to ask questions. Do not hesitate to ask your physician about possible side effects. If several medications are prescribed, be sure that you understand how frequently they should be taken. That is, should they be taken every day (prophylactic) or only when a migraine occurs (episodic)? Make sure you understand how frequently you may repeat doses in a given day and which medications may be taken together during a migraine attack.

You need to ask questions. Do not hesitate to ask your physician about possible side effects.

If your physician has ordered an MRI or CAT scan, make sure you understand the procedure. Let your physician know if you are claustrophobic, as you may need sedation for the MRI. Find out when you will be able to obtain the test results and how to get them (i.e., do you call the office for results or wait for your next visit)? See Questions 42 and 43 for more on MRI.

Finally, before you leave the physician's office, be absolutely certain that you understand when your return visit will be or if you need to call and make an appointment. In the latter case, be sure that you understand at what interval the return visit should occur or if it should happen only if you are experiencing problems with your migraines. Also, identify the office's policy regarding patient phone calls. Many offices have times set aside for physician phone calls, and finding out this information will make it much less frustrating if you know when the doctor is available. Do not be offended if you call your physician with questions regarding a medication or side effect and a nurse or physician's assistant returns your call. Many physicians have staff to assist them with routine calls, enabling them to focus on the patients in their office. These providers are trained to **triage** calls and problems for the physician. Of course, if you feel that you must speak with the physician, it is always appropriate to ask to do so.

Triage

The process of determining priority in treating patients.

Sometimes bringing a significant other who is familiar with your migraines and their effects on your life to the visit is helpful in both providing a complete history and remembering what was discussed. This approach has some disadvantages, however. Many patients find it difficult to discuss their pain and concerns openly in front of family members. In many cases, individuals feel guilt and shame associated with not being able to "handle" a headache. The relationship with the significant other may also be associated with other stressors that may not be freely discussed with that person in the room. Clearly, the choice of including another person in the discussion is a personal decision that needs to be made by the individual. A good rule of thumb is that if your practice is to take your significant other to all medical visits, then you will probably feel more comfortable doing so when you see a physician for your migraines.

If you do not, there is not a particular need to do so, at least for your first visit, unless specifically asked to do so by the physician.

46. What are clinical trials, and how can I participate in one?

Cherie's comment:

I highly recommend getting involved in a clinical trial if you meet all of the criteria. For me, I never would have made contact with my wonderful neurologist if I had not answered an ad for a clinical trial.

During your visit to the doctor's office, you may be asked if you would like to participate in a **clinical trial** to test a new medication or treatment approach to migraine. There are several ways in which a medication for a specific disease can make its way to the public. All drugs are studied by scientists and physicians before they are marketed to the medical world for patient use. New medicines are tested on animals for efficacy (whether it is beneficial) and safety, usually for years before they are tried on humans. Once they have passed the rigorous standards of the Federal Drug Administration (FDA) for safety and are ready to be tried on humans, the medication or regimen is tested in clinical trials.

Clinical trial

A research study used to test a new medicine or treatment for a disease.

For patients, clinical trials are often an opportunity to participate in groundbreaking research and try the latest options medicine has to offer. Nevertheless, clinical trials may or may not be an option for you. In some ways, it depends on the kind of person you are. If you like to be the first person to try something new or have interest in helping doctors learn more about migraine and ways to help yourself and other patients, clinical trials may be right for you.

Clinical trials offer the following advantages:

- Access to new medications
- Medications usually provided at no cost to those in the trial
- Close follow-up and access to study personnel during the trial
- Knowing the risks and benefits of all treatments, because they are laid out in writing prior to treatment
- The good feeling one gets from making a contribution to science and humanity

Clinical trials also have some disadvantages:

- Some trials are **blinded-placebo-controlled**. This means that you may be assigned to a group that receives a placebo instead of the real medication (placebo-controlled), and neither you nor the researcher will know if you are taking a placebo or the real medication (blinded). Keep in mind that a person's response to placebo is a biological phenomenon; it does not imply that his or her symptoms are not real. Some patients are not willing to join a clinical trial if they might potentially receive a placebo.

- The treatment regimen is determined by the research protocol as opposed to a totally individualized treatment plan.

- You may get started on a newly developed medication and feel well, but then the study might stop. You may not have access to the medication when the trial ends if the medicine is not approved for marketing and distribution.

Blinded-placebo-controlled

When setting up clinical trials, researchers prefer to compare treatments using a blinded-placebo controlled trial. This involves assuring that neither the patient nor the researcher knows whether the patient is receiving the actual medication or a placebo.

When you see your physician, ask about clinical trials if you are interested in pursuing this option. You may also visit the websites for the National Headache Foundation (*http://www.headaches.org*) and the American Council for Headache Education (*http://www.achenet.org*) to explore the availability of clinical trials in your area.

PART THREE

Migraine Across the Lifespan

How common is migraine in children?
Is migraine different in children than in adults?

Why does it seem that women have more
migraines than men?

What happens to migraine during pregnancy?

More . . .

47. How common is migraine in children? Is migraine different in children than in adults?

Migraine is seen throughout childhood and can begin as young as three years of age. The prevalence of migraine ranges from 1% to 3% in children younger than age seven and up to 11% from age seven to puberty. Prior to puberty, migraine is more commonly seen in boys. This finding is reversed following puberty, when migraine predominates in girls.

The criteria for diagnosing migraine in children are very similar to those used in adults; however, some of the more atypical types of headaches are more often seen in children. Also, the headache need not last as long in a child as in an adult to warrant a diagnosis of migraine. Children may present with dizziness and vertigo with vomiting as a variant of migraine. These children may be pale and unsteady. Intermittent abdominal pain that is without any other cause also may be a migraine variant. This type of migraine may be related to cyclical vomiting. All of these variants may occur in children of migraineurs, and these children may or may not go on to develop migraine with or without aura as teenagers or adults. Other children may have primarily eye manifestations of their migraine, with blurred vision and paralysis of the nerves and muscles controlling eye movements. In fact, children tend to manifest some of the more alarming variations of migraine, such as **hemiparesis** (weakness of one side of the body) and acute confusional state. It is important to rule out other more dangerous etiologies of these types of symptoms; if no other etiology is discovered, however, migraine may be the diagnosis of exclusion.

Hemiparesis

Weakness on one side of the body, usually the face, arm, and leg.

The evaluation of migraine in the pediatric population often begins with understanding the triggers and frequency of the headaches. This task may be particularly challenging in the younger child. An effort is made to appreciate the home and school situation and any potential stressors as well as to obtain a careful family history.

Working up alarming symptoms to rule out more serious neurological disorders is very important and will often reassure the concerned parent. Once psychosocial issues are appreciated, triggers identified and monitored, and other lifestyle issues addressed, pharmacologic management may be initiated.

The pharmacological treatment of migraine in children is similar to that of adults, with perhaps a greater emphasis on the first-line use of nonsteroidal anti-inflammatory drugs (NSAIDs). Triptans are often used in lower doses in the pediatric population. When these drugs have been studied in children, they appeared to have good safety and efficacy profiles. Many pediatricians and pediatric neurologists are comfortable using them because NSAIDs are quite effective in alleviating pain in these children. Because many children experience abdominal symptoms with their migraines, antinausea medications—which help both the headache and nausea—are often prescribed.

Preventive medicines are given to children as well. These medications are generally the same as those given to adults. Commonly used medications include valproic acid (an anticonvulsant), amitriptyline (an antidepressant), and propranolol (a blood pressure medication [an antihypertensive]). All of these medicines are effective in preventing migraine. As with all medications given to children, dosages are adjusted to their size and age.

48. Why does it seem that women have more migraines than men?

It is true that women have more migraines than men. A relatively steady 5% to 7% of men are migraineurs throughout the lifespan (**Figure 7**). The number of women migraineurs outstrips the number of men migraineurs by their early twenties, however, and the prevalence in women gradually climbs to more than 25% during the perimenopausal years. The overall prevalence of migraine is 18% for women and 6% for men, considering all age groups.

Both boys and girls may develop migraine before puberty. Girls are more likely than boys to become migraineurs during adolescence, a difference believed to be due to the onset of menstruation and the many hormonal changes that take place during puberty. At one time, migraines associated with menstruation, pregnancy, and menopause were all felt to be psychological, but now they are known to be neurobiological.

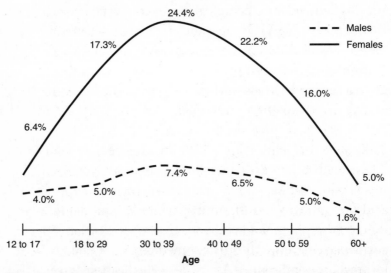

Figure 7 Prevalence of migraines by age and gender, according to the National Headache Foundation. Data are from 1999.

The relationship of ovarian hormones to the risk of migraine is an area of intense study. While the specific interactions and their effects on any given woman are not clear, researchers believe that the withdrawal of estrogen at the end of each cycle precipitates this kind of migraine.

More than 50% of women migraineurs report an increase in their headaches around menstruation. Usually these migraines are not associated with an aura, even if the woman has migraine with aura at other times of the month. Some studies show that menstrually related migraines are more severe and more difficult to treat than those occurring at other times of a woman's cycle. Other studies suggest that this may be true only for women who already have severe enough migraine to seek treatment. Fortunately, regardless of which category you may be in, treatment regimens geared toward specifically treating menstrually related migraine are available.

Three types of approaches are used in the treatment of menstrually related migraine. The first two are similar to the approaches used for all migraines—acute abortive treatment and preventive treatment. For menstrual migraine, neurologists often use short-term preventive therapy. This approach uses triptans every day during the two days before a period and during the first three days of a period. Studies have shown this method to be effective in reducing menstrual migraine. Nonsteroidal anti-inflammatory drugs (NSAIDs), may also be more effective during this time. Early studies using the new combination pill of sumatriptan and naproxen sodium indicate that using a triptan and an NSAID in one pill may also have a benefit in preventing menstrually related migraine. Finally, estrogen creams and patches used in the same fashion may confer some protection from menstrual migraine.

Many women notice that oral contraceptives (OCs) worsen their migraines. In fact, beginning OCs often precipitates a woman's first migraine. Others find that their headaches improve after starting an OC. If you wish to use OCs, you will need to work closely with your gynecologist and neurologist to find the best option for you to use. Switching to another OC may decrease the frequency of your migraines if they are particularly frequent, but the headaches may not disappear completely. Perhaps you will need to consider another form of contraception if all OCs worsen your headaches. Another option is to use a traditional preventive medication to decrease your migraine frequency. Your doctors should keep in mind the interactions between OCs and preventive medications when choosing the best regimen for you.

49. What happens to migraine during pregnancy?

The changes that women see in their migraines during pregnancy vary widely, and much research has focused on this issue in recent years. Several general themes have emerged, from both research and clinical observations.

Women who experience migraine without aura in the years before pregnancy, especially related to their menses, tend to have fewer or no migraines during pregnancy. This is thought to be due to the placenta producing increasing amounts of estrogen as the pregnancy progresses. Usually the headaches are worse during the first trimester but then dissipate during the second and third trimesters as estrogen levels increase. It is very important that you tell your physician if you are planning on getting pregnant so that you may plan your course of treatment together should you conceive.

For some women, their migraines actually worsen during their pregnancy. Migraines that were easily treated with over-the-counter medications may become unbearable during pregnancy, for example. If you have this experience, tell your obstetrician immediately. Usually you will be referred to a neurologist for evaluation to make sure that the headache is, in fact, a migraine and to begin a course of treatment to alleviate your discomfort. See Question 30 for more on treatment of migraine during pregnancy.

Unfortunately for the migraineur, the headaches usually recur in the postpartum period. These headaches may or may not be similar to the usual presentation seen prior to pregnancy, but given all the changes that a new baby may bring, one might expect that some components might be worse than others, or the headache might differ from pre-pregnancy migraines. The important thing to remember here is that some dangerous causes of headache are related to the postpartum state in women. These causes are varied and best evaluated by your obstetrician and a neurologist.

The best rule of thumb is that outlined in Question 17 for the dangerous headache. Dangerous headaches are defined as those that differ from any other headache experienced before; sudden, severe onset of any headache; onset of headache accompanied by loss of consciousness; headache associated with fever, stiff neck, and/or chills; gradual worsening of a headache; or change in the character of a headache. Adventitious (spontaneous) movements or twitching that appears to be seizure-like in nature also should send you to the emergency room immediately. Blurred vision or double vision may be ominous in the postpartum period as well.

The causes of dangerous headaches in the postpartum period are very rare. Our goal of presenting this information here is to educate you on what to look out for—not to alarm you. If in doubt, call your physician, describe your symptoms carefully, or have a family member help you. Spell out your concerns. You are your own best advocate in this situation. Should you not be able to reach your physician and your headache is worsening or otherwise alarming you, go to your nearest emergency room.

Some women have their first migraine during pregnancy. These migraines are usually migraine with aura, the type that is associated with lights and scintillating visual symptoms (jagged lines or **fortification spectra** described in Question 9) and scotoma (areas of darkening of the visual field). It is not really known why these headaches begin during pregnancy, and many neurologists work up these headaches extensively. Some of these women go on to have migraine on a postpartum basis, but many experience migraine only during pregnancy. If you are one of these types of patients, it is important that you tell your obstetrician, request to see a neurologist, describe your symptoms carefully, and seek immediate medical attention for any type of focal neurological deficit or symptom that you experience.

It is generally believed that migraines before and during pregnancy do not increase the risk of poor outcomes in pregnancy. In other words, the incidence of fetal malformations, miscarriages, premature labor, and stillbirths are not believed to be increased in women with migraine.

Fortification spectra

A visual phenomenon with a jagged appearance that usually begins prior to the onset of migraine pain. It usually begins centrally and gradually moves outward until it disappears.

50. I have heard that migraine improves after menopause. Is this true?

Menopause is said to have occurred when periods have ceased for 12 consecutive months. There are two types of menopause. The first is the physiological menopause that most women go through. Physiological menopause occurs when women gradually notice an irregularity in their periods and a gradual cessation of them altogether. This may take place over some months to years and may be accompanied by a myriad of symptoms—for example, hot flashes or night sweats, forgetfulness or other cognitive problems, dizziness, insomnia, depression, itchy skin, vaginal dryness, headache, and moodiness. The second type of menopause is surgical menopause; it occurs when the uterus and ovaries or just the ovaries are removed. With surgical menopause, symptoms occur within hours to days if hormone replacement therapy (HRT) is not started. Surgical menopause will not occur if only the uterus is removed.

Some women find that during the perimenopausal period (3 to 5 years before menopause) and menopause, they can no longer manage their migraines on their own. It is not uncommon to begin treatment with a neurologist at this time or to worry that your worsening headaches are the harbinger of something more serious.

The biggest hormonal change that takes place during the onset of menopause is the fluctuation of estrogen levels. The absolute level of estrogens during perimenopause is higher as well. This combination of estrogen fluctuation and higher levels of estrogen may precipitate migraine in female migraineurs. Perimenopause and menopause also may trigger new-onset migraines in some women, although this is less common. Consequently, these women should be worked up for other causes of their headaches.

Surgical menopause may acutely precipitate a worsening of migraine. Unless the surgery is for cancer or another life-threatening reason, the potential for significantly worsening migraine should be taken into consideration when a severe migraineur is assessing the risks and benefits of a complete hysterectomy or oophorectomy (removal of the ovaries).

For the majority of women, once estrogen levels cease their fluctuations and become lower than premeno-pausal levels, migraines decrease in frequency and may gradually fade. If they do not, HRT may decrease headache frequency, although there is some evidence that headache relief is not as complete as that seen with physiological menopause. Headaches may, in fact, worsen with HRT. Recent studies have also linked HRT to cardiac disease, stroke, and certain cancers later in life. Therefore, many recommend that HRT for migraine should not be used unless there are other benefits to using HRT such as the reduction of severe symptoms of menopause (e.g., intolerable hot flashes, night sweats, and so on).

Menopause is a particularly troublesome time for many women with migraine, because headaches tend to worsen at the same time that they are experiencing many other uncomfortable symptoms. It is wise to con-sider seeking treatment for your headaches at this stage of life if you feel overwhelmed by your headaches and other symptoms.

51. Is migraine common in later life?

If you are older than age 65 when you experience your first headache, it is important that you consult with your physician to explore possible causes for the headache. Only 2% of all migraine begins after the age of 65. Therefore, a new-onset headache is less likely to be a migraine, and a more involved medical and neurological history and work-up may be performed to make sure that a dangerous or reversible cause of the headache is not present. Headaches that are caused by other diseases or medications are called **secondary headaches**.

As we age, we tend to add more and more diagnoses to our medical history. Many of the illnesses and diseases that afflict us may also give us a headache. Some of these diseases are neurological in origin, whereas others are **systemic diseases**, meaning that they affect many organs or organ systems. Examples include severe anemia (very low red blood cell counts), kidney failure and dialysis, sleep apnea, acute hypertension, and very high calcium levels in the blood (hypercalcemia), to name a few. Usually correcting the underlying problem improves the headache. This care, plus the administration of headache medications, may be helpful in alleviating headache pain.

Still other secondary headaches may be due to the medications you are taking to control these and other diseases. Medications that are implicated in causing headache include those that dilate blood vessels, such as nitrates (nitroglycerin and nitropaste), Viagra®, and Cialis®, to name a few. Other medications known to cause headache are steroids, proton pump inhibitors (used for gastric reflux), selective serotonin reuptake inhibitors (SSRIs, which may also help headaches), nicotinic acid,

Secondary headaches

Headaches due to a specific cause, such as tumor, stroke, or head trauma.

Systemic diseases

Diseases that affect more than one organ system, such as high blood pressure, diabetes, and renal failure.

and Fosamax®. Certainly this list is not exhaustive and is not meant to be. Even so, whenever you are given a prescription for a medication, you should discuss its side effects with the pharmacist. Although headache may be listed as a potential side effect, you may not necessarily experience headache. But if you do, you may wish to discuss trying an alternative medication within the same class of medications or a medicine that accomplishes the same task, but through a different mechanism.

You also may experience other common disorders that can lead to headache such as stroke, brain tumors, subdural or epidural hematomas (traumatic blood clots in the brain), and herpes zoster. Less common, but distressing nonetheless, are trigeminal neuralgia and temporal arteritis. Nevertheless, neurologists keep an eye out for these types of disorders when they see someone older than 50 years of age presenting with a new or evolving headache.

Stroke

Sudden or gradual onset of focal neurological deficits due to a blockage of blood vessels in the neck or brain, or hemorrhage due to high blood pressure.

Carotid artery

One of the large vessels in the neck that provides blood to the brain.

Strokes are well known to cause headaches both acutely and chronically. Two types of strokes are distinguished: ischemic and hemorrhagic. Ischemic stroke occurs when an area of the brain does not receive enough oxygen, usually because an embolus (a clot) from the heart or the large artery in the neck (the **carotid artery**) breaks off and blocks a blood vessel in the brain. Hemorrhagic stroke occurs when too much blood reaches an area of the brain, rupturing the vessel and pouring blood into the substance of the brain. This type of stroke is usually seen in people with chronically high blood pressure or very sudden increases in blood pressure such as are seen with ingestion of substances like cocaine. Hemorrhagic stroke results in a blood clot in the brain. Usually the most alarming manifestations of a stroke are the numbness, weakness, and/or speech difficulties that accompany it. However, both types of stroke may be accompanied by headache. If the stroke is large enough, patients may suffer from headaches long after the acute problem is over. Medications are usually prescribed to alleviate stroke-related headache. To learn more about stroke and ways to prevent stroke in yourself and your loved ones, access the following websites: *http://www.stroke.org*, *http://www.strokeassociation.org*, and *http://www.stroke-site.org*.

A neurologist will usually consider a benign brain tumor, called a **meningioma**, as a potential cause of migraine in older patients. Meningiomas are benign tumors that arise from the meninges, the tissue surrounding the brain. They usually cause headache and neurological problems by pressing on the brain itself. If you are older than age 45 or 50 with new or worsening headaches, the cause may be a meningioma. These tumors, which typically grow very slowly, are usually readily visible on CAT scans and MRI and are often easily removed surgically. Medications may be useful in managing meningioma-related headaches if no other neurological problems are present. The doctor also will look for other types of tumors, and may suggest that you have contrast dye injected during the CAT scan or MRI to better visualize the brain. While the risk of tumor remains low, the tendency by doctors to image your brain to rule them out goes up as you age, because the risk of migraine decreases so dramatically.

Meningioma
A relatively common benign brain tumor seen often in women.

Your doctor may also be concerned about a traumatic blood clot in the brain referred to as a **subdural hematoma**. These types of blood clots are very common and may cause headaches, confusion, seizures, and focal neurological deficits if they become large enough. You may recall an event such as a fall or minor car accident ("fender-bender"), or even a bump to the head by hitting a cabinet or car roof. Over days to weeks you may notice increasing headache

Subdural hematoma
A traumatic blood clot of the brain that is often chronic and may lead to secondary headaches and seizures.

Epidural hematoma

A traumatic blood clot of the brain that occurs soon after the traumatic incident and may be fatal if not treated.

Herpes zoster

A rash or painful area of the face or trunk; also called "shingles."

Vesicles

Small blisters seen prior to the pain of shingles.

Neuralgia

Severe pain or tingling in the distribution of a nerve.

Trigeminal neuralgia

The trigeminal nerve is the fifth cranial nerve that controls sensation of the face. Abnormalities in this nerve may lead to a disorder characterized by severe pain and tingling in the distribution of this nerve.

with no other discernible symptoms. In the setting of a minor head injury and subsequent headache in later life, this is enough to warrant a simple CAT scan to rule out a hematoma—that is, a blood clot pressing on the brain. Subdural hematomas are usually easily removed and may even spontaneously go away with no surgery. Certainly, if accompanied by confusion, seizures, numbness, or weakness, the headache must be evaluated in an emergency room immediately, and surgery is usually indicated.

If you are involved in a traumatic event where you hit your head and are normal following the event but then become abnormally sleepy and/or complain of severe headache or any other neurological complaints within hours, you should be brought to the emergency room immediately. These symptoms may indicate the presence of a blood clot called an **epidural hematoma**. These types of blood clots are faster growing than subdural hematomas and may be very dangerous.

Seen throughout the lifespan, but very common in later life is **herpes zoster**, better known as shingles. With shingles, you may have **vesicles** on your face, neck, or trunk. After they have healed, you may notice very bothersome pain in the same area. This pain, which is known as **neuralgia**, is usually deeply aching, tingling, and/or burning in nature. You may be given pills and/or creams to alleviate the pain.

Trigeminal neuralgia is seen in all age groups but tends to be more common in later life. Its symptoms usually consist of severe, jabbing pain when certain parts of the jaw are touched or while chewing. Your doctor may order an MRI to look for lesions compressing one of the nerves supplying the face. If you have trigeminal neuralgia, you may be given medications or offered more invasive procedures to alleviate your pain.

If you are older than age 50 and are experiencing headache, your doctor may consider a diagnosis of **giant cell arteritis**. This unusual disease is treatable, which is why it is included here. Also called **temporal arteritis**, this disorder is characterized by a headache usually felt over the eye and temple and may be accompanied by visual loss or dimming. The vessel that traverses the temple may be enlarged and tender as well. If you experience fevers, weight loss, and muscle pains with this type of headache pain, this disorder is referred to as **polymyalgia rheumatica**, and your treatment will be coordinated with a rheumatologist. The diagnosis is made using a simple blood test, and often a biopsy of the temporal blood vessel is taken. The treatment consists of steroids with long-term follow-up by both a neurologist and a rheumatologist.

The good news is that migraines decrease later in life; however, aging is a mixed blessing. Suffice it to say that you should see your physician early and carefully describe your headaches. If you are not a "headache person"—that is, if you have never had headaches before—you can expect to have a more extensive work-up than a younger adult. In all likelihood, this work-up will be negative, but it is important to rule out potentially dangerous or disabling causes of headache.

52. Do migraines ever go away?

The prevalence of migraine decreases markedly after age 60. It drops to 5% in older women and less than 2% in older men from 20% and 8% in their younger counterparts, respectively. If you are a woman who suffers from migraines associated with your menstrual periods, you may find that once the monthly fluctuations in hormones cease postmenopause, you will have fewer and fewer migraines. Many patients also report that the

Giant cell arteritis

An inflammation of the temporal artery, which runs across the temple near the eye. This condition may lead to pain, headache, and possible visual loss if not treated.

Temporal arteritis

A rheumatological disease seen in older adults characterized by tender arteries in the temples and vision loss (partial or complete). May be associated with polymyalgia rheumatica.

Polymyalgia rheumatica

A rheumatological disease characterized by weight loss, fever, muscle aches and pain, and on occasion, vision loss (temporal arteritis).

The prevalence of migraine decreases markedly in later life.

headaches they do have are simply not that bothersome and do not require much more than over-the-counter medications as treatment.

Cherie's comment:

Migraines have become the bane of my existence. I am not quite certain why they have been coming more frequently. I have a feeling that only God knows for sure, but even my prayers have not been answered as yet. It seems that they never come at a convenient time. It has gotten so that I am afraid to make future plans without worrying that a migraine will screw up my plans and in turn my husband's as well. Fortunately I am blessed with an understanding and compassionate man who sympathizes with me and allows me to do whatever it takes to rid this pain from my head. It is a horrible way to live, and even after suffering a heart attack, a second coronary blockage, and a bout with breast cancer, I must confess that it is the migraines that I find to be the most debilitating of all. My greatest wish is to wake up one day and realize that it has been such a long time since I have had a migraine that I cannot even remember the last one!

PART FOUR

Managing Your Migraines: Taking Control

Does it help to keep track of my migraines?

What is a migraine trigger?

Why is it important to identify my migraine triggers?
How can I better identify them?

More . . .

53. Does it help to keep track of my migraines?

Cherie's comment:

I recommend that you keep a record of every migraine. Make a special notation in your appointment book or agenda. See if you notice a pattern. For instance, some women experience headaches at the onset of their menstrual cycle. For me, even though I no longer experience a period, I notice a pattern of monthly migraines perhaps connected to my hormone levels because I am still premenopausal.

Simply recording the days and dates of your headaches is helpful.

Keeping track of your migraines is a very useful technique both before you see a physician and afterward. Before seeing a physician, it is helpful for you to track the headache episodes to see if they follow patterns that you may not have noticed before. Luckily, the experience of others before you is helpful in this regard. Throughout this book we discuss triggers to migraine. A recurring theme is that of a probability for migraine, with triggers eliciting the actual headache. Because migraine triggers are so predictable and are predictable across many types of people, calendars can be set up to record specific triggers, which then allows you to look for certain types of patterns.

Simply recording the days and dates of your headaches is helpful. As discussed in Question 67, "letdown" headaches may occur at the end of the week. These types of headaches may even occur midweek if the stressful portion of your week occurs early in the week. If Monday, Tuesday, and Wednesday are your busy and/or stressful days of the week, then Thursday may be the day on which you suffer from your migraines. Or, you may suffer from your letdown headache on the more traditional Friday night or Saturday morning. Such headaches may be due to a decrease in stress or, if your headaches are related to caffeine intake, may be related to missing your daily double latte.

54. What is a headache diary?

An essential step you can take to help identify your own set of migraine triggers is to keep a **headache diary**. A headache diary is a daily written record of events, foods, thoughts, and feelings that occur with a migraine episode. It is easy to forget exactly how many headaches you had during a specific period and what you were eating, doing, thinking, or feeling prior to the attack. A written record becomes a valuable tool in this regard. It is also very helpful to record what you thought, felt, or did during and after an attack to better understand your coping responses to migraines.

Headache diary

A daily written record of events, foods, thoughts, and feelings that is used to identify a person's migraine triggers.

In addition to helping you identify your migraine triggers, a headache diary may be of great help to your physician. Bring your headache diary and list of possible triggers to your appointments; they will aid your physician in making a proper diagnosis and help you tailor your lifestyle to avoid frequent headaches.

It is virtually impossible to avoid all potential triggers, because some may be unavoidable parts of your life. Ideally, though, you should be able to reduce your exposure to those triggers that are particularly problematic for you, especially during vulnerable times when you may be more susceptible to a migraine attack.

You can choose among many different ways to keep a record of triggers. An example of a headache diary can be found in the Appendix. You may want to buy a journal or small book with blank pages just for this purpose, or perhaps keep a chart on your computer that can be printed out before office visits with your physician.

When keeping a headache diary, it is important to pay attention to a number of factors:

- What were the date and time of the headache?
- How long did the headache last?
- What type of pain did it present (e.g., pressing, throbbing, sharp, dull)?
- What was the pain intensity rating (on a scale of 0 to 10)?
- What was the location of the headache (e.g., behind the eyes, back of neck, temples, right versus left side of the head)?
- Were there any other physical symptoms (e.g., nausea, vomiting, fatigue, visual aura)?
- What were the emotional symptoms (e.g., irritability, anger, sadness, anxiety)?
- How were you feeling before the headache?
- What were you doing when the headache began?
- What was your mood or stress level before the headache?
- Were there any major changes occurring in your life (e.g., changes in job, relationship, health, finance)?
- What foods did you eat during the 48 hours before the headache?
- What was your sleep pattern during the 48 hours before the headache?
- Were there any particular weather changes prior to your headache?
- If you are a woman, where in your menstrual cycle did the headache occur?
- Which medications did you take after the onset of the headache?
- Did the medications offer any pain relief?

- Which types of nonmedication interventions did you use (e.g., rest, relaxation techniques, breathing techniques)?
- Did these nonmedication interventions improve your pain or mood/stress level?
- What was your mood during and after the headache?
- What were your thoughts during and after the headache?
- Any other comments regarding this headache episode?

A headache diary tracks many features of a headache. While it may appear to be a daunting task, you will probably find that recording the events around several migraines provides fruitful information to help you begin to take control of your headaches. Of course, a headache diary is effective *only* if you use it to identify your triggers. Fill out your diary as soon as symptoms start, or as soon as you are feeling better. Once you begin to identify your possible triggers, the next step is to begin to eliminate them or reduce your exposure to them as much as possible.

55. What is a migraine trigger?

Most migraine attacks are brought on by a long and varied list of events or conditions—for example, eating certain foods, emotional stress, sleep changes, travel, or skipping meals. An important distinction to understand is that these triggers are not the initial cause of your migraine condition, but rather activate an episode in a person who is already prone to getting migraines. If you have been diagnosed with migraine headaches, you are predisposed to having an episode that can be triggered by the long list of potential activators.

How these triggers activate a migraine is not exactly known. One theory is that the migrainous brain is in a constant state of baseline neuronal excitation. When a trigger comes along, it sets off the chemical cascade described in Question 3.

One of the most important things you can do in the treatment of your migraines is identify your migraine triggers.

One of the most important things you can do in the treatment of your migraines is identify your migraine triggers so you will be better equipped to avoid them and help prevent attacks.

56. Why is it important to identify my migraine triggers? How can I better identify them?

One of the most important steps you can take toward reducing the frequency of your migraines is identifying your migraine triggers. Everyone is different, and each person has his or her own set of potential triggers. Your task is to identify your unique set of triggers. By learning what is triggering your migraine episodes, you can then take steps to avoid those particular triggers. Eventually, you may be able to reduce the frequency of your headaches, which will make your life easier, less painful, and less stressful. By keeping a record of which foods, emotional situations, physical activities, environmental factors, weather conditions, sleep changes, and other triggers cause you to have migraines, you can begin to see your own patterns of triggers and stressful factors. There are many ways to record which daily events, foods, and/or environmental factors are affecting your headaches. One of the most effective measures you can take is to keep a headache diary, as described in Question 54.

57. Will my migraine triggers always generate a migraine headache?

Not all triggers you learn to identify as problematic for you will always set off a headache. Whether you react to a trigger may depend on your overall stress level at that time in addition to your simultaneous exposure to other triggers. For example, you may notice that particular triggers—for example, drinking a glass of red wine or traveling on an airplane—activate a headache. However, there may be times when you have a glass of wine while flying and do not experience a migraine depending on your mood, the reason for your trip, whether you are well rested, and so forth. Migraines often tend to occur when a number of triggers occur simultaneously or when you happen to be in a vulnerable state because of high stress or major lifestyle changes. Often, it takes a combination of emotional, food, and environmental stressors to bring about the biochemical changes that result in a migraine.

> *Migraines often tend to occur when a number of triggers occur simultaneously.*

58. What is stress?

The term **stress** has become a prevalent part of modern life. Everywhere you turn, you are likely to read or hear about stress. You have probably heard that stress can trigger migraines.

Stress
The way our bodies and minds respond to emotional, physical, and environmental changes.

So what exactly is stress? Broadly defined, stress is the way in which we interpret and respond to the changes and demands in our lives. Many types of stress exist, including stress caused by emotional changes, stress caused by physical changes, and even stress caused by changes in the environment. Stress is our attempt at adjusting to some kind of change, and it is a normal part of life. Hans Selye, the physician who pioneered much of the important research on stress, said, "Without stress, there would be no life." Although a certain amount of stress is expected in daily life, severe or chronic stress can lead to many medical and psychological disorders, including exhaustion, high blood pressure, immune dysfunction, depression, anxiety, and sleep problems. Stress can also trigger many preexisting health conditions, including migraine.

Sources of stress include poor health, accidents or trauma, financial worries, marital or family conflicts, occupational or relationship difficulties, bereavement, and divorce. There are also psychological stressors such as anger, depression, or anxiety. In addition, stress is caused by daily events such as traffic, loud noises, crowds, and living in an unpredictable world. Some sources of stress involve positive events, such as getting married, relocation, or a new job. Stress is an everyday part of life. *How* we cope with and react to stress is what determines its effects on our health.

59. Does emotional stress play a role in migraine?

Emotional stress is a common precipitating factor of migraine episodes and other types of headaches.

Emotional stress is a common precipitating factor of migraine episodes and other types of headaches. In fact, in one way or another, stress plays a role in all medical problems, with approximately 80% of all health problems now considered to be influenced by stress. Chronic stress and intense emotional events are the leading causes of psychological triggers in migraine sufferers. Most migraine sufferers eventually are able to identify the emotional stressors that trigger a migraine. Often, migraines may worsen around times of transition in a person's life, such as graduation from school or college, marriage, divorce, new employment, or changes in work, family, or financial status.

Chronic stress can produce emotional and biological changes that can directly affect migraines. Physical changes that occur from chronic stress include inflammation, changes in **vascular** function or blood flow, and the release of brain chemicals that can alter the pain threshold. All of these changes (which will be addressed in more detail in Question 60) influence the onset and severity of migraines.

Vascular
Having to do with blood vessels.

Who can say that they don't experience emotional stress in some part of their lives? Stress is unavoidable, and everyone reacts to stressful life events in their own unique way. It is how we perceive and react to stress that is important and determines its effects on our emotional and physical health.

Table 3 lists common stressful events. These life events are ranked from top to bottom in order of the amount of stress they may potentially cause.

Fight-or-flight response

State of arousal characterized by changes governed by the autonomic nervous system that include an increase in muscle tension, heart rate, blood pressure, and breathing.

60. How does emotional stress trigger my migraine?

Through a complicated combination of changes that occur within the brain and body, it is becoming increasingly clear that stress can lead to more frequent migraines as well as more intense headaches when they occur. When people experience a high level of stress, their bodies go into the **fight-or-flight response**. This state of arousal is characterized by changes governed by the **autonomic nervous system**, including increases in muscle tension, heart rate, blood pressure, and breathing. This natural emergency

Autonomic nervous system

Includes the sympathetic and parasympathetic nervous systems that transmit nerve impulses from the central nervous system.

Table 3 Common stressors.

- Death of a spouse
- Divorce
- Marital separation
- Death of a close family member
- Personal injury or illness
- Marriage
- Fired at work
- Marital reconciliation
- Retirement
- Change in health of family member
- Pregnancy
- Sex difficulties
- Gain of a new family member
- Business adjustment
- Change in financial state
- Death of a close friend
- Change to different line of work
- Change in number of arguments with spouse
- Large mortgage
- Foreclosure of mortgage or loan
- Change in responsibilities at work
- Son or daughter leaving home
- Trouble with in-laws
- Outstanding personal achievement
- Beginning or ending school
- Change in living conditions
- Revision of personal habits
- Trouble with employer
- Change in work hours or conditions
- Change in residence
- Change in schools
- Change in recreation
- Change in church activities
- Change in sleeping habits
- Change in number of family get-togethers
- Change in eating habits
- Vacation
- Minor violations of the law

Adapted from *The Social Readjustment Rating Scale*. Developed by Holmes and Rahe.

response equips us to handle a potentially threatening event and is a very effective way to cope with emergency situations as our bodies mobilize for survival. However, for people who are under chronic job, health, financial, psychological, or relationship stress, this emergency response is often continually activated. In these circumstances, the nonstop activation of the autonomic nervous system can cause physiological changes that contribute to and prolong migraine attacks and other health problems. Many people today are living with chronic stress, which can take its toll on emotional and physical health.

Stress contributes to the muscle tension and tightness in the head, neck, and scalp that are found in tension headaches and also in many migraine headaches. This muscle tightness can produce considerable discomfort and pain. The pain is often followed by anxiety about the duration and intensity of the headache, which can prolong the cascade of changes in muscle tension and blood flow—which initially triggered the migraine—resulting in a difficult cycle of emotional stress and pain.

Some neurochemical changes (changes in certain brain chemicals or neurotransmitters) are also associated with stress and migraines. As noted earlier, the autonomic nervous system, which is involved in regulating stress in the body, is responsible for the fight-or-flight stress response. During this stress response, the brain releases chemicals called **catecholamines**, which can lower the pain threshold and result in the experience of more pain. The autonomic nervous system also regulates anxiety, fear, irritability, concentration, sleep problems, and depression—all of which are symptoms common to many migraine sufferers.

Catecholamines

Brain chemicals that lower the pain threshold and result in the experience of more pain.

133

This may sound a little overwhelming and leave you wondering, "What can I do?" You should understand that the fight-or-flight response to stress is not the *only* way to react to stress. Questions in this and the next section identify ways you can alter your response to stress, thereby preventing or at least minimizing the intensity of migraine attacks. Question 94 addresses how to induce the relaxation response, which is the physical and emotional *opposite* of the fight-or-flight response. Learning to evoke the relaxation response is essential in reversing and managing the effects of stress on your physical and emotional health.

61. What are some examples of emotional stress-related triggers?

As you can see from Table 3, the list of emotional triggers is a long one. You should identify (perhaps by keeping a headache diary, as described in Question 54) which emotional stressors or situations are potentially difficult for you. Everyone reacts to life challenges and life stress in their own special way. By identifying which emotional situations or stressors are potentially dangerous to you as migraine triggers, you can begin to modify and change behaviors as well as learn to cope more effectively with the unavoidable stressful events (and many are unavoidable!) in your life. Examples of sources of psychological and emotional stress are interpersonal conflicts; arguments with family members, friends, or work colleagues; the daily hassles everyone goes through; and the periods of adjustment during changes in school, work, finances, or health status. Getting married, divorced, having children, and parenting are all major potential triggers as well. We can also feel stress from the way we think, feel, or behave when we are experiencing pressure in life. Emotional stress is unavoidable, but learning new and better coping strategies can help you manage all kinds of stress.

62. Are there foods that cause migraine?

Foods are probably one of the biggest culprits in the family of migraine triggers. Food intake is another pattern that often can be discerned with a carefully maintained headache diary. Given that so many foods and food additives can lead to migraine, it is not surprising that a person can eat many foods that are triggers without even realizing it.

Foods are probably one of the biggest culprits in the family of migraine triggers.

One of the biggest offenders is caffeine. Caffeine is ubiquitous in our society. For example, it is found in foods, soft drinks, and (obviously) coffee and tea. With the proliferation of espresso shops, we are now drinking more coffee and tea than ever before. In women, as little as two cups of coffee can be too much caffeine from a headache perspective.

Caffeine is a potent constrictor of blood vessels, which allows it to serve as a painkiller (which is why so many over-the-counter migraine preparations contain caffeine). When you stop the caffeine, however, the vessels dilate—and the result is often a pounding headache. This is probably one of the leading causes of weekend or "let-down" headaches in migraineurs who forego their "cup of Joe" on the weekend. The caffeine in many prescription medications such as Fioricet®, Fiorinal®, and Cafergot®, to name a few, is believed to be the culprit in medication overuse headaches. Therefore, it is critical that you keep track of all of your caffeine intake and replace as much as possible with noncaffeinated beverages (like those eight

Do not stop your caffeine intake abruptly or you will experience a rebound headache.

Rebound headaches

Headaches that occur when a medication is taken daily to relieve pain and then withdrawn. The headache recurs with greater intensity due to the withdrawal of the medicine.

Amines

One of the building blocks of proteins. These substances have been implicated as triggers for migraine and are found in many foods that set off attacks.

glasses of water you always hear about!). Beware, though: Do not stop your caffeine intake abruptly or you will experience a **rebound headache**. Taper it slowly. Be sure to carefully check labels of all soft drinks, sports drinks, and even herbal supplements. Remember—caffeine is added to many things. It is important to decrease or eliminate it from your diet if possible.

The next most commonly cited culprits as migraine triggers are chocolate and aged cheeses. Many of us enjoy these two foods—perhaps too much for our own waistlines and health! But what is in these foods that is problematic? Both contain **amines**. The amines in many foods come together to make proteins, but those found in chocolate and cheeses are particularly troublesome. Tyramine is the amine in aged cheeses, of which blue cheese and cheddar cheese are the biggest offenders. It is very important that you keep track of the cheeses that you eat and record whether you have a headache afterward. If you have a question about whether a cheese is aged, most cheese shops will be happy to point out those that are and are not aged, and some can actually point out a few of the headache culprits!

Chocolate is usually more obvious as a source of migraines. Many migraineurs have figured out that if they eat a single bar of chocolate, they will develop a migraine of distressing proportions. The lure of chocolate is a powerful one, and eliminating it from your diet may be very difficult. The best solution may be to monitor your cravings and avoid consumption in settings with other triggers. You may also try various brands of chocolates, as not all chocolates are equal, and one type or brand may be better tolerated than another.

Many women crave chocolate around the time of their periods, but the consumption of chocolate and the changes in hormones could be a disastrous combination if you are prone to menstrual migraines. Strict avoidance of chocolate perimenstrually (around the time of your period) may be the only solution in these cases.

Another class of foods that cause migraine is processed or preserved foods, which often contain **nitrites**. Nitrites are chemicals that dilate blood vessels, which can lead to a painful throbbing headache. Foods such as hot dogs, cold cuts, salami, pastrami, sausages, and smoked meats and fish all contain nitrites. Processed and packaged foods are everywhere in our society, so it behooves you to be a careful label reader and scout out nitrites among the list of ingredients on all packaged food that you eat.

Nitrite (nitrate)

A potent vaso-dilator found in medications and many packaged and preserved foods, especially meats.

Citrus fruits have been implicated as triggers for many migraineurs. It is not known why citrus fruits trigger migraines, but it has been postulated that food sensitivity or allergy could be the cause.

The use of a headache diary will allow you to better identify food triggers. You may have a specific food trigger not mentioned here. The key is to identify your unique food triggers and curtail your intake of these foods.

63. What about alcohol?

Alcohol is well known for its capacity to cause a hangover headache. It is also well known for its role as a migraine trigger. Red wines, dark beers, brandies, and champagnes are the most likely to trigger a migraine, although for many migraineurs any type of alcohol might bring on a headache. As with any trigger, you may not get a headache every time you have a drink. Interestingly, vodka and other clear alcoholic spirits are believed to have the lowest potential for triggering migraines, although clearly the best solution for avoiding alcohol-induced migraine is to avoid alcohol altogether.

64. Does exercise make migraine better or worse?

Exercise is probably at once one of the simplest and least complicated ways to improve your health. There is probably no disease that exercise will not improve. Exercise is beneficial for its cardiovascular effects and its assistance in weight-loss programs. It leads to a sense of well-being and relaxation and improves sleep. Exercise increases serotonin, and as outlined in Question 3, low serotonin levels are thought to play a role in the precipitation of migraine. It also increases the production of endorphins, which are chemicals the body produces that reduce pain and enhance pleasure. It is believed that exercising on a regular basis, which increases the release of endorphins and serotonin, may decrease the frequency and severity of migraines.

Always check with your physician prior to starting any exercise program, and build up your routines slowly. We recommend to patients that they begin with a simple walking program with achievable goals. Do not overdo things by being overzealous.

Unfortunately, exercise may actually exacerbate a migraine if you exercise during the very early phases of an attack. Once you already have a migraine, exercise may make it worse. Even minor exercise, such as walking up stairs or carrying items such as groceries, causes vessels to dilate, and this in turn leads to the release of chemicals that initiate the pain cascade. Therefore, if you feel a migraine coming on, it is wise to not exercise. To decrease the risk of exercise-induced headaches, including migraines, you may also try taking ibuprofen prior to exercising. Indomethecin, which requires a prescription from your doctor, may also protect you against exercise-induced headaches.

If you feel a migraine coming on, it is wise to not exercise.

65. I have heard that the environment can play a role in triggering migraine. Is this true?

If you have noticed that the weather affects when you have a headache, you are not alone. Changes in barometric pressure and increases in humidity are two environmental factors that seem to trigger migraines. Bright sunlight and cold winds also are frequently mentioned as precursors of headaches or migraine, as are flickering fluorescent lights, pollens, molds, and solvents.

Be sure to scan your physical environment for potential triggers or you may miss them. While many of these factors may be beyond your control, knowing their potential impact is reassuring if you are troubled by an otherwise unexplainable migraine.

66. I take certain medications that seem to give me migraines. Is this common?

Medications are a big culprit when it comes to causing headaches. Many medications list headache as a potential side effect, and some medications are particularly prone to causing headaches. For example, medicines

139

that dilate blood vessels (nitroglycerin, Viagra®, Cialis®), treat depression (selective serotonin reuptake inhibitors [SSRIs]; see Question 74), relieve gastric reflux (proton pump inhibitors), and treat hypercholesterolemia are all known to cause headaches. Fosamax®, oral contraceptives, and steroids also may result in headaches in susceptible individuals. This list is by no means exhaustive, but merely demonstrates that commonly used medicines cause headaches. Of course, these medications do not cause headache in everyone who takes them.

At the same time, many medications that cause headaches might also relieve headaches. SSRIs are used in depression and have been associated with headaches and migraine. However, many headache specialists prescribe SSRIs for the preventive management of migraine. A similar phenomenon is seen with steroids. If used chronically, steroids may lead to headaches, yet short bursts of steroids may break a bout of severe migraine pain.

If you are on a medication that causes headache, your physician may change you to another medication within the same class of medicines (i.e., a medicine that works by the same mechanism) or to a medication that treats your medical problem but via a different mechanism. Another option is to keep you on the medicine suspected of causing your headache and also treat your headache. It is important that you discuss all these options with your physician, and that you understand the plan and how it will affect the management of your headaches as well as your other medical problems.

67. Why do I get headaches on weekends or on the first day of vacation just as I am beginning to relax?

It seems particularly cruel and ironic that just as you are beginning to wind down and relax at the end of the week or have just started that long-awaited vacation that you are hit with an intense migraine attack. Unfortunately, many people suffer from "weekend migraines," which are also called **letdown migraines**. These are just what they sound like—attacks that occur on weekends or just as you are starting to unwind from a busy work week. The triggers for these headaches appear to be tied to the eating, sleeping, and other lifestyle changes that often occur on weekends or vacations. They likely are related to the fatigue and exhaustion that are produced by a busy and stressful week, and to the vascular and neurochemical changes that may occur after an intense build-up of stress.

Letdown migraine

Migraine episode that may occur after a period of emotional or physical stress and that frequently occurs on weekends. Also known as a "weekend migraine."

Let's start first with some of the behavioral changes that usually occur around weekends. Frequently, when the weekend arrives, you may change your sleep habits by either staying up late or sleeping later in the morning (and possibly both). As addressed in Question 70, it is important that migraineurs establish consistent sleep patterns. Too little or too much sleep can serve as a trigger, because the changes in sleep may cause physiological and blood flow alterations that trigger migraines. Also, you may go longer without eating on weekend mornings or change your diet. Major changes in sleep, behavior, exercise, and diet are all potential triggers of weekend and vacation headaches.

Major changes in sleep, behavior, exercise, and diet are all potential triggers of weekend and vacation headaches.

Another key trigger in letdown or weekend migraines is that weekends may follow a period of extreme stress. Maybe you have found that after a particularly stressful week, you were hit with an attack. Other examples include working under extreme pressure for a week or longer in preparation for some major deadline, or perhaps a work or social event that you were responsible for planning, or a major holiday family function such as Thanksgiving or Christmas. After you've pulled off the event with flying colors, you get sidelined with a major attack. Probable causes are the physiological letdown effects after extreme emotional and physical stress, and the likelihood that you were on emotional overdrive during that time, possibly ignoring or avoiding the build-up of stress and pain. Ways to modify your emotions and behaviors to avoid or reduce letdown or weekend migraines are discussed in Question 68.

68. What can I do to help prevent weekend or letdown headaches?

The prevention of letdown or weekend headaches requires planning. The key to migraine control is the self-regulation of thoughts, feelings, and bodily functions. Of course, this is easier said than done! While it may be a difficult task, planning ahead to maintain balance can reward you by preventing an episode or reducing its severity.

One major trigger of weekend and letdown headaches is change in sleep pattern. The best way to avoid these changes on weekends is to set your alarm on the weekend morning at the time or close to the time you would get up during the week. This sounds a little unfair in that for many people one of the joys of weekends is "sleeping in" and trying to "make up" for lost sleep during the week. Paradoxically, this oversleeping can leave you more tired and may trigger a bad migraine attack. Try to be consistent in your sleep habits. You should apply these principles to vacations, too, though it can be difficult when traveling to different time zones. Question 69 provides information on travel as a trigger. Also, while on vacation or during travel, you may be sleeping on a bed and pillow that have a different firmness or texture than at home, causing changes in neck posture and tension. If you have a special pillow that reduces neck tension, you may want to bring it along. You can also practice relaxation techniques and neck stretching before sleep and upon waking in a different bed.

Be mindful of eating changes on weekends. Do you eat late on Friday? Do you indulge in extra sweets or alcohol that might be a trigger for you? Does your intake of caffeine change? Also, try not to wait too far into Saturday to have your first meal. Sleeping late along with not eating for a longer period of time can serve as a potential trigger.

Many migraine and tension headache sufferers share the problem of chronic or built-up upper back, neck, and scalp tension during the week that they often ignore. This tension might not be enough to cause you to feel debilitated, but it is enough to cause you a mild amount of pain or discomfort throughout the week. This annoyance usually goes ignored as you get through the week accomplishing work and social plans or goals. An unfortunate consequence of avoiding or ignoring this low-level headache and tension throughout the week is that when the weekend arrives and your stress level changes, you may be hit with a severe and debilitating migraine or tension headache.

As described throughout this book, it is vitally important that you prevent the onset of migraines through the use of various physical, emotional, and mind–body techniques *before* they happen. Instead of avoiding or trying to distract yourself from the pain and build-up of tension and stress you feel all week, be mindful of these changes and direct your attention toward them, rather than away from them. You can try one of the many relaxation or mind–body techniques described in Part 6. Mindfulness meditation is an extremely useful way to increase your awareness of these trouble spots and to learn to identify the links between thoughts, feelings, and bodily reactions. You can also have a massage at the end of the week or apply other strategies that may help to relieve the weeklong build-up of tension.

Prevent the onset of migraines through the use of various physical, emotional, and mind–body techniques before they happen.

69. Why do I frequently have migraine attacks when I travel?

Just as with the weekend or letdown headaches, people who get migraines find it particularly difficult and extremely unfair that when traveling on business or vacation they are struck with frequent and debilitating migraines. Many migraine sufferers experience a fear of travel because of their history of frequent migraines while away on vacations or business trips. The increased risk for having a migraine when traveling simply reflects the fact that when you travel, you expose yourself to an increased number of migraine triggers—specifically, changes in stress level, sleep pattern, time zones, mood, weather and altitude, diet, and general changes to your routine. Many of these changes or disruptions can occur quite suddenly.

Nothing is worse than not being able to enjoy the first day of your long-awaited vacation in a beautiful place. As with many of the strategies to minimize the frequency and intensity of your migraine, the solution is to be prepared and plan ahead. The rest of this question identifies some problem areas and solutions to minimize the chance of a migraine, so you can maximize your enjoyment while away.

Stress

Stress is a primary trigger of migraine, and planning for a vacation or a business trip is typically a stressful experience. For most people, leaving for a vacation usually follows a stressful period at work, school, or home as you hastily try to prepare while taking care of loose ends. This build-up and release of stress leaves you vulnerable to a letdown headache (see Question 67). It is also one reason why many people have a migraine attack while traveling or on the first day of arrival in a new location.

To avoid this problem, start planning early, and don't leave packing until the last minute. Don't make your last few days at work or school exceptionally stressful. Don't leave projects and deadlines hanging over you until the last minute. The typical rushed and stressful last few days prior to a vacation are a powerful migraine trigger.

On the eve of your travel, take time out to relax and wind down a bit. Practice some deep breathing and participate in some activity you find relaxing and enjoyable.

While traveling, practice relaxation techniques such as breathing exercises, playing relaxing music, or meditating. If you are traveling by plane or train, it could be the perfect place to practice your **relaxation techniques**.

Relaxation techniques

A wide variety of techniques, including breathwork, meditation, guided imagery, and yoga, to promote relaxation and physical and mental well-being. Used commonly in the treatment of stress and pain-related conditions.

If you are driving, take a break and let someone else drive so you can find some time to rest. If you are on a stressful business trip, it is especially important to practice forms of relaxation to combat the stress of your schedule. Even vacations can be stressful. Don't try to overdo things while traveling or sightseeing. Respect your body and don't push yourself. Slowly allow yourself to wind down while monitoring your emotional and physical reactions. The reward for being prepared and paying attention to stress will be an enjoyable vacation.

Medications

You might be surprised how many people either forget to take all their medications or deviate from their regular medication schedule while on vacation. Days before leaving a trip, check whether you have enough of each medication to take with you. You may want to ask your doctor if you should bring an additional amount since you'll be away. Keep all medications in their original containers with the name of the medication, your name, and the doctor's name on it. Never keep medications loose or unlabeled. In addition to possibly confusing you, this practice puts you at risk of having customs agents confiscate your pain medication. Take your doctor's telephone number with you.

Don't deviate from your regular medication schedule. If you are changing time zones, do your best to maintain a regular medication schedule. If you take medication for motion sickness, be sure to pack it in your carry-on prior to leaving.

Diet

When you are visiting some new place, it is enjoyable to experiment with different cuisines while you soak up the local culture. Even when on business or traveling within their native country, people will usually overindulge in sweets, eat too much, change their eating schedule, or change their alcohol or caffeine level. Be conscious of what you are eating and when you are eating. Don't stray too far from your routine schedule, and be mindful of your migraine triggers. If you know that red wine is a potential trigger for you, don't risk having a glass while you are already exposed to so many other different conditions and risk setting off a migraine. While traveling on long trips, be sure to drink plenty of water, and avoid the temptation to indulge in junk food that may be available.

Sleep

As has been said throughout this book, sleep is a vital area of concern for migraineurs. Unfortunately, many factors can disrupt your regular sleep pattern when you are traveling. The main challenges are trying to maintain your routine while traveling to different time zones, staying up all night while flying on an airplane, or experiencing sleep disruption due to the stress or excitement of traveling.

There are some situations you obviously cannot avoid. Even so, try your best to maintain a regular sleep schedule. If you are flying overnight, try to sleep during the flight. Perhaps your physician can help with a sleep aid. Do not drink alcohol while flying to try to make you sleepy. In addition to being a trigger for many people, alcohol does not promote a restful sleep and contributes to dehydration. Be prepared for a change in your sleep environment once you arrive at your destination, including the firmness of the bed, room noises, or uncomfortably hot or cold rooms.

If you are struck with a migraine, however, do not catastrophize it by saying to yourself, "Now the whole vacation is ruined!" Instead, practice all the techniques you have learned and put them into action. If you need to, take time out and be alone. While others may be saddened that you are not able to join them on a particular event, it is important that you take care of yourself to shorten the length of the attack so you will be able to get back on your feet soon. Try to maintain a positive outlook with a self-statement such as "Losing one day out of two weeks won't destroy this vacation."

Finally, try to maintain as regular a schedule as possible. With enough preparation, you can minimize the chance or severity of a migraine while allowing yourself to enjoy your travel experiences.

70. I have trouble falling asleep on a regular basis, which seems to make my migraines worse. Are there any steps I can take to improve sleep?

Sleep disorders are a major problem for migraineurs, just as they are for the general population. More than half of all Americans report a history of insomnia or some other sleep disturbance at some time during their lives. While sleep problems may cause distress and health troubles for anyone, they are particularly problematic for those suffering from migraine and other pain disorders. Insomnia or other sleep disturbances often trigger a migraine episode, while having frequent migraines makes it difficult to fall asleep. This may result in a vicious cycle in which headache and other migraine symptoms prevent you from sleeping while the lack of sleep further perpetuates migraines. Making an already difficult situation even more complicated and confusing is that sometimes sleep can be the remedy for a migraine, but other times it can also be a trigger.

Undoubtedly you have experienced times when you were feeling exhausted, irritable, and uncomfortable from a migraine episode, and all you wanted to do was sleep. You finally try to fall asleep, but find that the stress, pain, and generalized discomfort make it impossible to do so. Unfortunately, the stress and anxiety of not being able to fall asleep make it even more difficult to sleep, further intensifying your pain and stress level.

Symptoms of insomnia or sleep problems include:

- Having a hard time falling asleep within an hour of going to bed even when you are very tired
- Having a hard time staying asleep throughout the night
- Having frequent early-morning awakenings (waking up between 3:00 and 6:00 A.M.) and not being able to fall back asleep
- Even when getting a full night's sleep, not feeling rested upon awakening

Although migraine is clearly linked to sleep disorders, other medical conditions can be the cause of insomnia. If you are experiencing severe sleep problems, report this fact to your physician. People with severe sleep problems will sometimes undergo an evaluation at a sleep center or with a sleep specialist. A chronic lack of sleep is also associated with depression and anxiety disorders, further complicating an already complex and challenging situation. One possible reason for the overlap between sleep problems, migraine, and depression is that all these medical problems are believed to be associated with the regulation of the brain neurochemical **serotonin**. People who suffer depression or anxiety will experience more depressive and anxiety symptoms due to sleep deprivation; at the same time, depression and anxiety frequently result in an inability to fall asleep. Once again, this results in a frustrating cycle. Although these difficult cycles are challenging to break, the following questions outline steps you can take to improve your sleep pattern and consequently reduce the frequency and severity of migraines.

Serotonin

A neurotransmitter involved in the regulation of moods and pain.

71. Are there any changes in my diet or medication that could help improve my sleep?

This book has frequently mentioned the relationship between sleep and migraines. Clearly, many sleep disturbances can profoundly affect migraine and, conversely, migraine can produce sleep disruption. The following are some general guidelines related to diet and medication that may improve your sleep situation.

Avoid stimulants at least six hours before bedtime. This includes all drinks or foods that contain caffeine, such as coffee, cola, tea, hot chocolate, or chocolate. You also may want to avoid foods or drinks that contain high amounts of sugar late at night if you believe you are sensitive to them.

Avoid alcohol late at night. In addition to being a migraine trigger, alcohol can disrupt healthy sleep cycles, resulting in a less restful sleep. Although alcohol may cause you to feel sleepy and relaxed at first, it has adverse effects on your sleep. While alcohol may help put you to sleep, many people find that they wake up earlier than expected when the alcohol wears off.

Be aware of medications that can disrupt sleep. Some medications act as stimulants, including pseudoephedrine (a common decongestant), diet pills, caffeine-containing prescription drugs, and some other drugs used to treat a variety of medical problems. Speak with your physician to see if the medications you are taking can affect your sleep.

Avoid going to bed too full or too hungry. Don't eat heavy meals after 7:00 P.M. The process of digestion and the full feeling you experience can make it more difficult to fall asleep or sleep soundly. However, don't go to bed so hungry that you can't sleep.

Beware of a reliance on sleep medications. Your medical doctor may prescribe sleep medications for you. Be sure to talk with the neurologist or physician treating your migraine about the appropriate way to use these medications. Although medication for sleep can be helpful in the short term, it can result in additional sleep problems if used for too long a period. Drugs that aid sleep are useful if you are going through an emotional crisis or stressful time, or perhaps are traveling to a different time zone. Chronic use of these medications, however, can result in a reliance on them to sleep or cause a "rebound" effect, making it more difficult to fall asleep. Although these medications may work in the short term, they do not address or resolve the underlying reasons for sleep disturbances.

72. What else can I do to improve my sleep habits?

In addition to paying attention to what you eat and what medications you take, it is equally important to develop good sleep hygiene and habits while eliminating the habits that may be contributing to the problem.

Use the bed for only two things: sleep and sex. If you have trouble falling asleep, avoid the habit of using your bed to read, do paperwork, talk on the phone, or watch TV. This helps to train you to associate the bed with only the two activities of sleep and sex.

Keep a sleep diary. Just as you record all events and your diet in your headache diary, record how much sleep you are getting each night, and notice whether it has any relationship to the onset of your migraines. Things to record include what time you go to bed, what time you wake up, how long you sleep, and how you feel in the morning.

Keep a regular sleep schedule. Try to go to bed the same time every night and awake the same time each day. Maintaining a sleep routine with the same amount of sleep each night is essential to achieving proper sleep hygiene and reducing sleep-related migraines. Review Questions 67 and 68, which deal with weekend and letdown headaches. Remember, oversleeping can be a primary trigger for migraines. If you are short of sleep one night, don't try to "make up" for it by sleeping late the next night or on weekends. Sometimes a short sleep can end a migraine attack, but at other times it can initiate one. Learn what works for you and what your sleep triggers are by keeping a sleep diary.

Find ways to relax. A common reason for sleep problems is anxiety or a racing mind, so learn ways to relax before going to bed. Begin to wind down in the early evening so you don't have to switch from a very active physical or psychological state to a restful one in a short time. Apply some of the many relaxation techniques described in Questions 94 through 98. Simple breathing techniques or the body scan technique can be very helpful in reducing muscle and emotional tension prior to bed. Perhaps a warm bath will work for you.

If you can't sleep, don't stay in bed. If you find yourself twisting and turning and getting frustrated that you can't sleep, get out of bed and do something passive such as light reading and then return to bed when feeling sleepy. Don't go to bed unless you are tired. You can't force sleep! Trying to sleep when you are worried about not sleeping will just make it harder to sleep. Don't be so hard on yourself: Take a break. Return when you are tired.

Exercise during the day. Exercise is an excellent way to improve sleep, reduce physical and psychological stress, and improve your overall health. However, don't exercise immediately before bedtime. Leave at least 6 hours between exercise and bedtime so you are not too stimulated by the workout to be able to sleep. Exercising in the morning is a wonderful plan if your schedule permits it. Be sure to read Question 64 on exercise and migraine.

Create a sleep-friendly environment. Make sure the temperature, the mattress, and the noise level are comfortable for you. Put time into making your bedroom a calm and soothing place for sleep and rest. You might want to have a CD player on your bedside table so you can play relaxation CDs. Don't make your bedroom your office. Do all your work in a different place than the bedroom.

Keep a positive outlook. Even if you think you can't sleep, try to avoid making self-statements such as "If I don't sleep, I'll perform horribly at work tomorrow" or other catastrophizing comments. Don't "clock watch" all night. Try to keep things in perspective. When you are overtired, your coping skills don't stay as sharp. Remember all of the things you can do to improve your sleep. Say to yourself that losing sleep tonight won't be the worst thing in the world.

More information on sleep-related issues can be obtained by contacting the National Sleep Foundation. Information for this organization is in the Appendix.

PART FIVE

The Emotional Side of Migraine: Learning to Cope

I've been feeling increasingly depressed and anxious.
Is there a connection between depression,
anxiety, and migraines?

My doctor prescribed an antidepressant medication
for me. Does this mean that my migraines
are caused by depression?

I find myself struggling with emotions such as
anger, guilt, and shame.
Are these types of feelings common?

More . . .

73. I've been feeling increasingly depressed and anxious. Is there a connection between depression, anxiety, and migraines?

Many migraineurs at some point in their life experience anxiety or depressive symptoms. In fact, migraine patients are more likely to experience clinical depression or anxiety than people without migraine or headache disorders. Research indicates that 34% of migraine sufferers will experience depression at some point in their lives compared to 10% of people with no history of migraines. Migraine sufferers also have a greater chance of having an anxiety disorder than nonmigraineurs, with 54% of migraine patients having an anxiety disorder at some point in their lives versus 27% of those without a migraine history. Migraineurs are more likely to suffer from panic attacks, sleep disorders, and other psychological problems. Often these problems may coexist.

Everyone at some time experiences feeling blue or down in the dumps. Occasional sadness and anxiety are normal parts of life, especially if you are struggling with a chronic pain condition such as migraines. Clinical depression or anxiety disorders, however, are more than just occasional episodes of feeling down—they are long-lasting mood disorders that can lead to problems in work, relationships, and health. Clinical depression can impair a person's ability to function in many areas of living, and if severe and untreated can lead to suicidal thoughts or actions.

Although the relationship between migraines and depression is complex, we'd like to point out three important ways that these two medical problems are linked. The first, and maybe the most obvious, is that people who live with chronic pain conditions such as migraines are more at risk for depression, anxiety, and other psychological problems because of the suffering they experience secondary to their migraines. Migraine patients often feel forced to alter their schedule, often canceling social, work, and other planned activities. Additionally, because of frequent or intense migraine episodes, you may begin to experience changes in your relationships with family members, friends, or work partners. Consequently, the suffering that accompanies migraines can lead to social withdrawal, further complicating your ability to maintain the quality of your relationships. Isolating from others during difficult periods is a risk factor for depression. Changes in sexual functioning, concentration difficulties, sleep changes, and feeling hopeless in the face of repeated migraines all place a person at risk for anxiety and depression. Because depressive feelings may cause further isolation and can even lead to more increased headache frequency, it is imperative that the depression be treated.

A second reason why migraineurs might have higher rates of depression is because both depression and migraines involve changes in certain brain neurochemicals, particularly **neurotransmitters** called norepinephrine and serotonin. Serotonin is among a class of neurochemicals believed to play a major role in the regulation of mood and pain. Depression and migraine sufferers both share a reduction in serotonin levels in the brain. This neurochemical vulnerability predisposes a depressed patient to migraines *and* a migraine patient to depression. Low serotonin levels can cause vascular changes and dramatic alterations in blood flow in the brain. This is the reason why your physician may have prescribed antidepressant medications that regulate the levels of serotonin in the brain (as discussed in Question 74).

Neurotransmitters

The chemical messengers in the nervous system. These chemicals are involved in pain, emotion, mood, sensation, movement, and the special senses.

Depression and migraine sufferers both share a reduction in serotonin levels in the brain.

157

Other effects of low serotonin are fatigue, decreased sex drive, sleep disturbance, and chronic pain conditions other than headaches.

A third potential connection between migraine and depression and other psychological disorders is that a history of depression, anxiety, trauma, or other psychological or psychiatric disorder may predispose a person to headache disorders as well as other pain and health problems. One explanation is that people with a history of depression or other psychiatric disorder may have neurochemical changes that make them vulnerable to migraine and other problems. Also, having a past emotional crisis or extended periods of distress may result in difficulty coping with severely stressful conditions. It may alter how your body reacts to stress. This increases the likelihood of depression and anxiety when confronted with a health problem later in life. This does not imply a weakness on your part or any reason for blame, but rather a biological and psychological vulnerability to stress and potential emotional suffering. If you have had a history of depression, anxiety, trauma, or physical or sexual abuse, it might be very beneficial to consult with a mental health professional.

In summary, there is a relationship between depression, anxiety, and migraines. Many researchers and mental health professionals believe they are similar in that they are all neurological reactions to severely stressful conditions. A history of depression increases the risk of migraines, and, conversely, a history of migraines can place you at risk for depression. In addition, severe migraine problems can mask or hide an underlying depression. Further information on how to determine if you are depressed and where to seek help are in Questions 74 and 75.

74. My doctor prescribed an anti-depressant medication for me. Does this mean that my migraines are caused by depression?

There are a couple of reasons why your doctor has prescribed an antidepressant medication. One of the primary reasons doctors prescribe this type of drug is that many of these medications target the same neurotransmitters of the central nervous system that regulate the onset of migraines. As discussed in Question 73, it is believed that serotonin (a neurochemical in the brain) is directly involved in both the regulation of mood and the amount of pain you feel. Two classes of antidepressants, **tricyclic antidepressants** and **selective serotonin reuptake inhibitors (SSRIs)** regulate these serotonin receptors that appear to be the brain's major pain regulators (see Question 19 for more information about medications).

Since a primary biological cause of migraines appears to be a disruption of serotonin levels in the brain, antidepressants are a first-line offense as a preventative migraine medicine. Common tricyclic antidepressants used for prevention of migraine are amitriptyline and nortriptyline. Some examples of SSRIs are Fluoxetine (Prozac®), Paroxetine (Paxil®), and Setraline (Zoloft®). A significant number of migraineurs take antidepressant medication to maintain appropriate levels of serotonin that will aid in the prevention of attacks. Taking an antidepressant medication for migraines doesn't mean the doctor thinks your headaches are a symptom of depression or are not real. Your migraine pain and the depressive feelings they can sometimes cause are *both* real.

Tricyclic antidepressants

A class of antidepressant medication also used to treat headache and other pain conditions.

Selective serotonin reuptake inhibitors (SSRIs)

A class of antidepressant medications that regulates the neurotransmitter serotonin in the brain.

The relationship between depression and migraines is complex. In addition to antidepressants being used to target brain chemicals that regulate pain, migraineurs may also suffer from depressive or anxiety disorders. You may have experienced changes in your mood as a reaction to living with migraines. Clearly, the emotional changes that migraines put you through can bring on sad and depressed moods as well as changes in sleep. Sometimes the consequences of severe and/or frequent migraines can result in a depressed mood that lasts more than the occasional difficult day and may last weeks or longer. If this is the case, you may find that antidepressants prescribed by your doctor may relieve these symptoms as well as your migraines.

You should feel comfortable to ask your doctor what the medication you are prescribed is for. Don't be reluctant to ask for details about the medications you are taking and what the objectives are. The more you know about your own treatment, the more empowered you will feel as a participant in the relief of your migraines.

75. How do I know if I am depressed?

Occasional or periodic experiences of sadness or "feeling blue" are a normal part of life. These are natural reactions to the challenges, changes, disappointments, and losses everyone goes through. Patients who struggle with the physical and emotional challenges of migraine and other pain conditions report higher rates of depression than the general population. Depression is a major healthcare problem affecting roughly 15 million Americans. One of the crucial things to understand in the context of migraines is that chronic depression can place you at higher risk for a migraine disorder and for more frequent and intense migraine attacks.

So, how do you determine if you are clinically depressed or just struggling with transient sad moods as a reaction to migraines and other life stressors? It is common for migraineurs, particularly those experiencing frequent attacks, to become discouraged, hopeless about receiving effective treatment for their migraines, to increasingly feel sad, and to socially withdraw from their regular social and occupational activities. If you find that you are avoiding activities, spending more time alone, and finding less enjoyment in the things you once enjoyed, this may indicate a depressive disorder. If you find that you have a sad mood most of the day for more than two weeks at a time, feel hopeless about the future, experience a loss of energy or appetite, have changes in sleep, and an inability to concentrate or remember things, then you are clearly struggling with some of the primary symptoms of depression. Feeling overwhelmed and having thoughts of suicide are serious symptoms that require immediate attention.

You may sometimes think that you are alone in your reaction to your migraines. The truth is that you are not alone. Many people do suffer depressive disorders, and feeling sad or depressed most of the time is *not* something that should be ignored. Some people might respond, "You're going through so much with your migraines, of course you're going to feel down some days." You may have had past difficult times in your life where you experienced stress and emotional suffering, but you came through that experience within a reasonable period of time. If you find that your mood changes are lingering and you experience the symptoms listed in Table 4, you owe it to yourself and your loved ones to seek professional treatment. The good news is that depression and anxiety, when properly diagnosed, are treatable disorders. Remember, how well you cope with your migraines and the emotional suffering they cause has to do with your being an empowered participant in your treatment.

Depression or anxiety can sometimes manifest as physical symptoms in addition to emotional complaints. Some examples of physical symptoms are weight loss or gain, decreased sexual drive, body aches or pain, and fatigue.

Tables 4 and **5** list some criteria for depression and anxiety disorders. Review these lists. If you can identify with any of the items, let your physician know to determine whether a consultation with a mental health professional is indicated. These lists are not intended to replace a professional consultation, nor do they allow you to make a self-diagnosis. Specific medical conditions can mimic these symptoms. Only a qualified professional can make a diagnosis of depression or anxiety disorder.

Questions 77 and 78 provide information on when and whom you should consult with if you decide to seek help. A number of organizations provide information to the public on mental health and illness and are listed in the Appendix.

Table 4 Symptoms of depression.

- Depressed mood nearly every day, tearfulness, feelings of emptiness
- Diminished interest or pleasure in activities you previously enjoyed
- Poor appetite or overeating, weight decrease or increase
- Sleep disturbances (increase or decrease in sleep; frequent awakening)
- Low energy or fatigue
- Poor concentration or difficulty making decisions
- Feelings of hopelessness or excessive guilt
- Low self-esteem
- Recurrent thoughts of death, or thoughts or plans of suicide

---

Derived from *Diagnostic and Statistical Manual of Mental Disorders* (DSM-IV)

Table 5 Symptoms of anxiety.

- Excessive anxiety and worry for most days
- Restlessness or feeling on edge
- Frequent fatigue
- Poor concentration, mind going blank
- Feelings of irritability
- Muscle tension
- Sleep disturbances (difficulty falling or staying asleep, restless sleep)

Derived from *Diagnostic and Statistical Manual of Mental Disorders* (DSM-IV)

76. I find myself struggling with emotions such as anger, guilt, and shame. Are these types of feelings common?

Migraineurs often experience a broad range of emotions, including anger, guilt, and shame as well as other difficult feelings. This is often made worse by fears and assumptions that people think you're lazy, are avoiding work or relationships, or are using headaches to seek attention. It is normal *and* common to experience difficult emotions when struggling with a chronic medical problem, depression, or negotiating a major life change. Other common feelings and psychological symptoms that migraine patients report are hopelessness about the future, feelings of emptiness or low self-worth, fatigue, depression, and anxiety. If these feelings become overwhelming, it might be necessary to seek help from a licensed and qualified mental health professional such as a social worker, **clinical psychologist**, or psychiatrist. A history of depression or other psychiatric problems can predispose one to various pain conditions. Conversely, migraine and other pain conditions may predispose a person to depression. You may benefit from the help of a mental health professional as you try to understand the feelings you are having.

Clinical psychologists

Specialists in the science of mind and behavior. They have a doctoral degree and provide various forms of psychotherapy and other clinical interventions to treat a wide variety of mental health and emotional disorders and concerns. Psychologists are not medical doctors and do not prescribe medication.

163

In the wake of repeated headaches and missed social or work appointments, you may begin to think that you are inadequate, that somehow you cannot tolerate the pressures of life as others can. Feelings of self-blame or shame are common but unrealistic. Migraines are a neurological disorder and, although your specific coping style may alter your pain threshold, it did not cause you to have migraines in the first place.

It is also common to experience anger. You might be angry with yourself for having repeated attacks; at family members for not better understanding, helping, or supporting you; or even angry with them because you believe that they don't believe you. You may be angry at life, or if religious, angry with whatever your belief in God is for allowing you to suffer. Or perhaps you are struggling with anger related to other circumstances in your life. Remember that anger is one of the emotions that can have a powerful effect on migraine pain, as it often increases the pain level. The impact of anger on migraines and other health problems is a serious and widespread health problem. Anger results in a release of brain chemicals such as adrenaline that can profoundly affect health. Some of the physiological consequences of internalizing anger include muscle tension, teeth grinding, constriction of blood vessels, increased heart rate, high blood pressure, and flushing of the face. All of these bodily reactions often serve as triggers to migraine headaches. Prolonged or bottled up anger can lead to neck and jaw pain, headache disorders including migraines, high blood pressure, heart attack, and stroke among other medical problems. We have all heard the common sayings associated with severe anger such as "My blood is boiling" or "I'm so angry that I'm seeing red." Medical science is now beginning to grasp the enormous impact of emotions such as anger on health.

However, anger in itself is not a dangerous emotion. Actually, the healthy expression of anger is a key factor in good physical and psychological health. Everyone feels anger. It is *how* we deal with anger that is important. Unhealthy expressions of anger include bottling it up or internalizing it, misdirecting it, or emotionally escalating to the point you often feel out of control. A healthy way of dealing with anger is to address what is causing you to feel angry before it builds up to unhealthy levels. Once you recognize what is making you angry, you can directly speak with the person or persons that might be involved, or find ways to address the problem that is causing distress. This can be combined with practicing effective coping techniques such as "taking time out," physical exercise, or practicing one of the many relaxation techniques described in this book such as relaxation breathing, meditation, or creative visualization.

A healthy way of dealing with anger is to address what is causing you to feel angry before it builds up.

Although it is common to experience emotions such as anger, guilt, or shame, it is essential that you learn ways to feel more in control of them than feeling they control you. Allow yourself to feel whatever emotions are coming up for you, and do not internalize or avoid them. Speak with someone you feel comfortable with or seek out professional help. Try to keep a diary of your feelings and thoughts. When feeling overwhelmed, try to incorporate the relaxation techniques outlined in this book. Know that you are not alone in your migraine pain. Question 80 provides information on finding support groups or organizations that understand what you are going through.

77. When should I consult with a mental health professional?

There are many instances when a person suffering with migraines or other headache disorders could benefit from seeking treatment from a mental health professional. If you were able to identify with many of the symptoms of depression and anxiety provided in Question 75, a consultation with a mental health professional could prove helpful and is recommended. Feeling sad or anxious for long periods of time, getting less enjoyment from life events or relationships, or having recurrent thoughts of hopelessness about the future all are indicators that you are struggling with complex and difficult emotions. Thoughts of death or suicide require immediate medical and psychiatric attention. Being alone often makes these feelings worse. As you likely know, it is sometimes difficult to address these hardships with family members, a spouse, or friends.

A consultation with a mental health professional offers a safe and confidential place to address these issues. A professional will help you identify the reasons why you are feeling depressed or anxious, and through a close working relationship, the therapist and you will collaboratively reach appropriate methods for addressing and solving the problems that may seem insurmountable at first. This may be achieved through **psychotherapy** or through the use of medication, referred to as **psychopharmacotherapy**. Sometimes these two approaches are combined, and there is excellent evidence that when individuals are suffering from severe or long bouts of depression, the combination of the two approaches proves extremely helpful.

Psychotherapy

A term used to describe a wide variety of talking and behavioral therapies to treat a variety of mental health and emotional conditions and disorders. Used to treat depression, anxiety, and adjustment concerns related to stress and relationships.

Psychopharmacotherapy

The science of using medication to treat psychiatric disorders, conditions, and symptoms.

Depression and anxiety are treatable conditions. Unfortunately, people are often reluctant to seek help for psychological conditions such as depression or anxiety because of the stigma that is frequently associated with mental illness. Depression and anxiety, just like migraines, are health problems that can be treated. There is no reason to experience shame concerning depression any more than any other health problem. Fortunately, the stigma over psychological and psychiatric disorders is lessening; however, it is often still difficult for many people to reach out for help. If you have had a history of depression, anxiety, problems with alcohol or drugs, or have undergone physical or sexual abuse or some other form of trauma, talking to your doctor about getting a referral to a mental health professional is highly recommended. Remember, consulting with a mental health professional does not mean that the migraines are "all in your head." Seeing a mental health professional is very useful in dealing with the *real* emotional reactions to living in chronic pain. Many patients report feeling relief and an enhanced sense of control soon after beginning treatment. *It all comes back to taking control and empowering yourself as an active participant in your health.*

Another primary reason why you could benefit from treatment with a mental health professional is to learn better ways to effectively cope with the challenges of migraines. You could choose to do this at any time. Mental health professionals who work with migraine patients and other individuals struggling with medical problems are experts at teaching effective methods to experience increased control over migraines and stress. You will also learn and practice coping strategies that will aid in dealing with the unpredictability of living with migraines.

Depression and anxiety are treatable conditions.

78. What type of mental health professional should I choose?

Choosing a mental health professional requires many considerations. First, you need some information on what types of professionals offer the type of care you may need in the behavioral treatment of your migraines as well as the treatment of any psychological or mood disturbance you may be experiencing. The person you select should be licensed to practice in your state and should have the appropriate degree and qualifications to practice his or her specialty. Secondly, it's important to feel comfortable with the person you've chosen. Getting "the right fit" is one of the most important steps in selecting a therapist. Take time in assessing the chemistry between you and this person. Do you feel comfortable with him or her? Can you talk to her about any personal or private matter? Does this person create a comfortable environment and treat you in a respectful way? Do you feel that the therapist is really effectively listening to you? These are some of the questions you should ask yourself. Feel free to interview different therapists. Also be sure to ask the mental health professional if he or she has experience working with patients diagnosed with migraines.

The following is a list and description of mental health professionals who are most qualified to address your emotional difficulties:

Clinical Psychologists: These are specialists in the study of mind and behavior who hold a doctorate in clinical psychology. This can either be a PhD (Doctorate of Philosophy) or PsyD (Doctorate of Psychology). A clinical psychologist specializes in the diagnosis and treatment of a wide range of psychological and behavioral disorders in children, adolescents, and adults. They provide clinical services to individuals, couples, families, and groups. Examples of problems they treat are depression, anxiety, marital conflicts, drug or alcohol addiction, low self-esteem, and relationship problems, and they also help individuals adjust to difficult periods of transition in life. Clinical psychologists are trained in various types of psychotherapy. Examples are psychodynamic, cognitive, and behavioral. It is ideal to find a therapist who works in an integrative style incorporating each of these schools of therapy. Feel free to ask the psychologist what type of therapy they offer. Clinical psychologists who specialize in health psychology or behavioral health are often experts in providing relaxation and stress reduction techniques, and are trained to work with medical patients including individuals with migraine and other chronic pain conditions. A doctorate-level clinical psychologist must have a license to practice in your state. Clinical psychologists do not prescribe medication, but work closely with psychiatrists who do prescribe, and they can refer you for medication if indicated.

Psychiatrists: These are medical doctors (MDs or DOs) who upon completing medical school continue their education to specialize in treating mental, emotional, and behavioral disorders. Since psychiatrists are physicians, they are experts in prescribing medication for the treatment of disorders such as depression and anxiety. Many psychiatrists also provide psychotherapy or work with clinical psychologists. Psychiatrists who work in the field of consultation/liaison psychiatry or psychosomatic medicine have additional training in treating patients with health problems including migraines and other chronic pain disorders. A psychiatrist must have a medical degree from an accredited medical school, have completed a residency program, and be licensed to practice medicine in your state.

Clinical social workers

Professionals who provide a wide range of social and supportive services in hospitals and other health settings.

Clinical Social Workers: These are professionals who have received a master's or doctoral degree in social work (MSW, DSW, PhD) and offer a wide range of social and supportive services in hospitals and other health settings. Many clinical social workers or psychiatric social workers are also trained in providing psychotherapy or counseling services. Clinical social workers require a state license to practice.

Clinical psychologists, psychiatrists, and clinical social workers provide services that are reimbursable in part by your health insurance. Check with your health insurance provider to determine what the mental health benefits are for your plan.

79. Should I take psychiatric medications to help with the way I feel?

If you are feeling severely depressed, anxious, or are experiencing sleep problems, trying medication to alleviate or improve the condition could prove very useful. As discussed in Question 74, many of the medications used for depression also help in the treatment of migraines. If your doctor thinks you might benefit from a psychiatric medication for a particularly emotionally difficult period, or if you are thinking of this type of treatment, you should consult with a psychiatrist who specializes in the use of medications.

80. Are there other forms of support I can get?

Aside from professional resources like physicians and mental health professionals, there are also other places to receive support for your migraines. Often, a combination of many approaches will provide the best results.

Most migraine sufferers find it very helpful to know that they are not alone in their suffering, and it often feels comforting to be around others who are going through the same physical and emotional changes. One place to find this type of support is with local support groups. The bonds that are formed in support groups made up of people who have migraines can be extremely beneficial. Being around people who understand your situation is often a very valuable experience. Aside from receiving support and a "good ear" in a support group, you may also learn about techniques or strategies that have been effective for other people. Sharing of helpful hints or effective therapies can also be a useful function. There is scientific evidence that people who attend support groups often feel better, experience more control in their lives, and may actually improve in their medical condition.

Most migraine sufferers find it very helpful to know that they are not alone in their suffering.

Support groups for migraine and headache patients can be found by contacting national migraine and headache resources or local mental health professionals who specialize in migraines, or individuals can form them on their own. Your local school, religious organization, and community center all are good places to start your search. The Appendix lists some national resources.

81. What can I do to better cope with my migraines?

Living with chronic migraines is a difficult and challenging experience. It is common to feel a host of complicated and difficult emotions, and often feel helpless in your struggle against migraines. One of the most common complaints that migraine and other headache sufferers express is that they have little or no control over their migraines or the events that initiate them. Feeling you have no control over life events can be a frightening emotion. Unfortunately, this only makes you feel worse and can even increase your migraine pain. It is important to know that there are steps you can take to feel more in control and improve your ability to cope. No matter how difficult things get, there are measures you can take and resources you can contact for help. Just by reading this book and consulting some of the resources listed, you have already taken a step toward feeling more in control of your migraines versus being a victim of them.

Everyone copes with life problems in different ways. Coping involves a very individualized set of behaviors and responses that are unique to each person. No two people cope in exactly the same way. The essential goal is to find the coping strategies that will help you manage *your* pain and stress satisfactorily. One of the first steps to take to improve coping with migraines is to learn how you are currently reacting or coping. Sometimes, individuals with chronic migraines or other pain conditions develop ways of coping that may in fact be maladaptive and lead to increased pain. This is likely not your intention, but is an unfortunate and common occurrence. *How we perceive and experience our pain will have a direct effect on the pain itself.* In other words, our emotional reactions to a migraine headache can either potentially produce an *increase* or *decrease* in pain intensity depending on our type of reaction.

One common but ineffective way of coping is to avoid or ignore the problem. Yet, ignoring the problem or the stress it creates will not make it go away. Another common response is to have negative, self-defeating thoughts. Sometimes you may find you catastrophize a situation by thinking to yourself, "This is the worst headache I've ever had," or, "This headache will never end." Other examples are thinking you will lose your job, impair relationships, or need to go on disability. While all of these consequences are of real concern to you, it is more likely that one particular migraine episode is not the worst of your life, or that it will not last forever. Thinking the worst scenario results in you feeling more anxious, frightened, depressed, and out of control. When stuck in this type of thinking, it becomes very difficult to make good decisions and deal effectively with your migraine headache. By having an anxious and panicked response at the start of a headache, you might bring about the severe headache that you were afraid of in the first place. This type of hopelessness may actually delay your taking medications in a timely fashion if you tell yourself, "nothing ever works."

Learning to replace catastrophizing or self-defeating thoughts with more realistic or positive statements is a key step toward effective coping. Instead of thinking this headache will be the worst ever, make the statement, "Although it feels very bad, I know it won't last forever and I should not panic." Try to practice some of the relaxation techniques in this book, take time out, or even write off part of the day and vow to return to whatever you were doing when the headache is over.

There are many factors involved in learning to cope more effectively with migraines, many of which are outlined throughout this book. The following is a brief review of some of the ways you can improve your strategies to cope with migraines:

- **Monitor and decrease emotional stress**. By learning the various relaxation methods outlined in Questions 94–97, you can develop ways to reduce stress and alter your response to stressful situations. A few minutes of focused breathing can be surprisingly helpful. If spirituality plays an important part in your life, draw upon your spiritual practice or spiritual community for support, strength, and wisdom. Meditation, prayer, or reading spiritual or philosophical books that are important to you all can be helpful in keeping things in perspective. Humor is also a very effective stress buster! Although there is nothing funny about migraine suffering, try to maintain a sense of humor about things when you can.

- **Exercise and stay active**. Exercise is a great way to both reduce emotional and physical stress and improve overall health resulting in less headache and other medical problems. Be sure to read Question 64 on migraines and exercise. Stay active and try to keep a regular routine as best you can. Modalities such as Yoga, Tai Chi, and the Feldenkrais method are all excellent movement modalities that include stretching, strengthening, spiritual, and relaxation components as part of the experience. You can learn any of these at classes offered by yoga centers, gyms, spas, or community centers.

- **Identify migraine triggers**. By using a headache diary or other type of headache journal, you can identify and eventually avoid exposure to potential migraine triggers.

- **Change your emotional reaction to migraines**. Migraines often result in catastrophizing emotions with accompanying statements like, "This headache will never go away," "I will never get better," or "These migraines are going to cause me to lose my job or my relationships." Learn ways to reframe a migraine episode by making statements that are more realistic and positive.

- **Get support**. You are not alone in your migraines. Millions of people suffer severe headaches. Reach out to support groups and the many headache societies and organizations listed in the Appendix of this book. Try not to isolate. Speak directly and honestly about what you are going through to family and friends if you believe they can be supportive.

- **Be prepared with medication**. Always have medications with you in case of an attack. Comply with the medical plan outlined by your physician.

- **Seek professional mental health help if necessary**. If the emotional roller coaster of migraines is taking a toll on your ability to enjoy life, then reach out to a mental health professional to address feelings such as depression, anxiety, guilt, shame, anger, and other difficult emotions. A qualified professional will also help you identify sources of stress and teach you effective coping and relaxation techniques. Refer to Question 78 for more information on mental health professionals.

- **Learn to express emotions and set limits on what you can do**. Learn effective ways to express yourself. Learn to say "no" to demands you just can't do. Set limits with your time. By working with some of the steps presented in this book or by working with a licensed professional, learn how not to bottle up or internalize emotions such as anger, sadness, resentment, or disappointment.

It is important to remember that neither your migraine headaches nor the way you deal with life's struggles developed overnight. Effective coping takes time and persistence. By beginning to think and react differently to migraines, you have already begun taking control.

82. My migraine headaches are having a negative impact on my relationships with my spouse and family members. What can I do to improve this situation?

One of the most distressing effects of migraine headaches is the impact on family and marital life. Migraines can potentially affect every aspect of family living, causing profound changes in the emotional and social environment of marital and family life. Frequent migraines may alter your ability to carry out your role as mother, father, brother, sister, or spouse in the way you would like. Family events with children or important social engagements with your spouse may have to be canceled due to an intense migraine episode. Again and again, you may feel as though you have ruined another chance for your family or for you and your spouse to have quality time together. This may result in your experiencing guilt as well as sadness, disappointment, or anger that in turn only contributes to the intensity of your headache. This can leave you feeling both physically and emotionally terrible. Although these experiences are distressful, as with any conflicts or trouble spots in relationships, they also can afford the opportunity for a stronger connection with the important people in your life. Sustaining a healthy marriage and family life in the face of migraines is surely a challenge; however, there are effective ways to identify what the problems are and make way for improvement.

Because the effects of migraines can frequently disturb the family or marital routine, they are also frequently at the center of many conflicts. If these conflicts continue without mutual understanding and direct and honest communication, they can wreak havoc on any marriage or family. Occasionally, everyone in the family experiences sadness, loss, anger, blame, frustration, or guilt for the missed opportunities and the stress of living with chronic illness. Often, family members keep these emotions to themselves, causing difficult emotions to only intensify, which can contribute to feelings of resentment. The following are some steps to help you and your family cope in a better way:

- **Educate family members, spouses, and partners.** Don't assume they understand what you are experiencing. Your family is likely confused and not quite sure what to do when you have a migraine. Their attempts to help may in fact irritate you more. Pain is a very personal and subjective experience. When you are not having a migraine, sit down with your spouse, children, or family members and educate them on what you experience during a migraine. Give them reading materials if you think that will help. They can read it on their own time and likely get a better sense of the physical and emotional roller coaster that can sometimes characterize the migraine patient's life. Show them this book or alert them to the many resources listed in the Appendix. Inform them that migraines are a legitimate medical and neurological disorder. It is important to be patient, direct, and honest. Be careful not to appear judgmental or resentful if at first they don't understand. Dealing with your migraines is likely a confusing and difficult situation for them as well as you.

- **Separate the migraine problem from other family problems.** It is important not to let family, relationship, or communication problems be "masked" by problems linked with your migraines. If there are conflicts related to how much time is spent together as a family, financial concerns, or parenting responsibilities, for example, it is extremely important not to fall into the trap of blaming the migraines for these conflicts when they have been problem areas all along. Don't allow yourself or family members to "use" migraines as the reason for unrelated conflicts.

- **Don't allow migraines to be your identity**. Having migraines is clearly something that you experience; however, it is extremely important to recognize that *your migraine pain is not you*. What do we mean by this? Often individuals with chronic pain or headache conditions begin to feel as though pain is part or all of who they are. Try to think of the suffering that pain causes to be just something you pass through—only a temporary episode. It always does eventually pass. *You and your pain are separate*. If you begin to view pain as a permanent aspect of your personality, it becomes difficult to cope. Remember, *you are not your pain*. You may experience suffering, but the suffering is not you. Question 94 on meditation further clarifies this point.

So if you begin to see yourself as assuming the identity or role of a migraine sufferer, remember that your identities such as father, mother, husband, wife, and so on are your primary life roles. When you are migraine-free or on a day that you can function better, do your best to assume and enjoy these roles. Family members will likely relate with you better when you have migraines if they see you as vitally engaged in family activities when you are feeling better. Don't allow all family conversations to center around your migraines.

83. Sometimes I feel as though family members, friends, or coworkers think I am being manipulative through my migraines. What can I do about this?

This is a good and important question. Often we hear that migraine sufferers as well as individuals dealing with other chronic pain conditions worry that family members, friends, or coworkers might think they are complaining of migraines to get out of work, receive attention, or benefit in some other way. Maybe a family member or someone has even accused you of this during an argument.

Although you would never dream of having a migraine to get something from others, it is important to understand how migraine pain can sometimes cause complicated behaviors on the part of the migraineur. Although a person couldn't imagine getting *something good* from their migraine pain, it may in fact be possible that they do receive some benefits while in pain. During a severe episode, you might be aware that others help you out by taking over your responsibilities for a while or that you are excused from family functions or events. Perhaps you are "allowed" to take time off while others have to somehow make up for your absence. While not implying that you consciously intended to get pain for these reasons, it is important to recognize if you do receive some benefits when you are feeling sick. An honest examination of how your migraines affect others and yourself is essential. This may necessitate an honest conversation between you and family members or your spouse.

Psychologists sometimes refer to the benefits received while impaired as secondary gain. While you may not be consciously aware of seeking out these rewards, it's important to recognize that this can and often does occur. This is not a reason to blame or evoke guilt in the patient, but it does provide an opportunity to determine if a migraine sufferer has "learned" that he or she may receive certain rewards when sick. If this goes unaddressed, the risk is that these behaviors can evolve into a pattern where a person derives certain actions from others through migraine pain versus learning to directly ask for it. This is sometimes a difficult idea to accept, and again, this is not a reason for self-blame. Remember: *You didn't choose this migraine.* A migraine is a result of complex physiological actions in your brain. However, take a careful look at how people respond to you when you are having a migraine. If upon examination, you think it is possible that you do receive certain responses and benefits from others that you perhaps couldn't directly ask for, take this opportunity to acknowledge and learn ways to change these behaviors. It all comes back to not allowing migraines to control your life and behaviors, but at best, to provide an opportunity to better understand and even empower yourself while learning to manage and cope with migraines.

84. Migraines have had an effect on sexual intimacy. How can I address this issue with my spouse or significant other?

When migraines are frequent and a chronic part of life, the desire for and pleasure of sex can often be compromised. If you are feeling physically and emotionally exhausted, sexual activity is not likely an attractive option to you at that time. The cycle of migraines and loss of sexual intimacy may cause you to feel less desirable or to withdraw from your relationship. You may become less communicative while at the same time harboring many emotions. Often, this can result in one or both partners feeling angry, hurt, rejected, resentful, confused, or unsure of how to change things.

Chronic migraine pain does not mean that your sexual life should be diminished. Despite migraine attacks, with effective communication and honesty, you can still maintain a healthy and satisfying sexual life. As with any sexual and intimate relationship, it is imperative that both partners be direct and honest with their feelings. Although it might seem obvious to you that sexual activity during a migraine episode isn't appealing, your partner may be hurt when you decline his or her sexual advances. You may wonder, "How could I be desirable with the way I feel and look?"

Silence will not help at all. However, the best time to speak about this issue is *not* when you are having a migraine but at some other time when communication will be easier and emotions aren't so loaded. Be direct and inform your partner that when you are experiencing a migraine, you cannot enjoy or have sex. Reassurance that this is unrelated to other hidden feelings and that you are not angry or sexually turned off is important. Don't assume your partner knows what you are going through during a migraine. Explain that sometimes you might be irritable or easily annoyed and that these too are symptoms of feeling so miserable during a migraine attack. Educate your partner or spouse about your needs and your limitations during an attack.

If your sexual desire and ability is diminished not only during a migraine attack but also over a longer period of time, then an examination of possible causes is needed. If you think medications are affecting your sexuality, speak with your doctor. For men, some of the medications prescribed may have an impact on the desire or physical ability for sexual intimacy. Your doctor can alter your dose or change medications to resolve this adverse effect.

Other causes can affect sexual desire or performance. Underlying or unresolved emotional problems in your relationship can manifest in your sexual relationship. If one or both partners are experiencing unaddressed emotions such as anger, hurt, or rejection, these emotions can often be consciously or unconsciously expressed in the bedroom. Also, a loss of sexual desire or ability can be the result of other medical (gynecological or urological) and/or emotional problems. If you think this may be the case, you should speak with your physician and consider consulting a mental health professional who works with couples, such as a clinical social worker, psychologist, or psychiatrist. Questions 77 and 78 describe the various mental health professionals who practice psychotherapy.

85. As the loved one of a migraine sufferer, I often have a difficult time coping with my family member's migraine. What can I do to better cope and be of more help?

Max's wife's comment:

My husband has headaches, both migraines and regular everyday headaches. He almost never complains about them—actually, he just about hides them from me. He will tell me about a headache after he has had it for a day—and that may only be the midway point. But sometimes he needs to lie down and sleep. I do not get angry, but I do feel helpless. It's not his fault, and he is the one suffering. I also feel guilty when I know he has a headache and we go about our daily lives. I know that he doesn't feel 100% and that he may be pushing himself for me.

It is well known that migraines can have a serious effect on family members and spouses, and that family members may in fact experience the same emotions that the migraine sufferer feels. Spouses, children, parents, and significant others of migraineurs all may experience emotions such as guilt, sadness, loss, anger, and helplessness. Allow yourself to acknowledge that having these emotions is a *normal* part of living with someone with a chronic illness. In recent years, the healthcare community has begun to get a clearer sense of how much chronic illness impacts others in the family. Some general guidelines to be aware of are:

- **Take time to care for yourself.** Just as we advise the migraineur to be clear with others about their needs and limitations, so should you. Set reasonable expectations on what you *can do* for your loved one as well as what you *cannot do*. Take time to nurture yourself during or after stressful periods. Practice some of the relaxation techniques described in Questions 94 through 96. If you find that you are having a difficult time with the complex and challenging emotions that living with a migraine sufferer can sometimes bring, you might want to think about consulting with a licensed psychotherapist to help you deal with your burden. Question 78 outlines what types of mental health professionals are available.

- **Ask the migraine sufferer what you can do to help**. When your family member is migraine-free, ask them what you can do when they are experiencing a migraine. Ask them to name their expectations. You may think that by saying, "Don't let this migraine ruin the day. Let's go to the movie anyway; you'll feel better when you get there," that you are helping when it might only anger your family member. Ask them what helps and what you should and shouldn't say. They may prefer you to be around and offer support. Conversely, they may want to be left alone and not talk at all.

- **Don't minimize the suffering caused by migraines**. Living with someone with a chronic pain illness is challenging. Be aware of tendencies (these are normal too!) to get angry and minimize your family member's misery. They are doing the best they can and feel guilty enough on their own. Minimizing their pain or blaming them won't help matters.

- **Communicate**. Although living with chronic illness in the family is a challenge, it also provides a chance to solidify and deepen your relationships. A by-product of these challenges can be an opportunity to experience a greater sense of compassion and love. If you have strong feelings, tell them to your family member on a day when he or she is migraine-free.

86. My migraines are affecting my performance at work. Are there any strategies that I can use in the workplace to cope better?

Just as migraines can profoundly affect your relationships with family members, loved ones, and friends, headache pain also can have a major impact on your ability to perform well in the workplace. In fact, the impact of migraine on the workplace is enormous, costing the economy billions of dollars each year in lost workdays and unemployment. Roughly 10% to 20% of migraine sufferers are unemployed due to the hardships of living with migraines, an unemployment percentage higher than that of the general United States population.

People who suffer with chronic migraines often experience difficulty negotiating the demands of work, worry about missing too many work days, have trouble maintaining adequate concentration to work efficiently, or feel that their relationships with coworkers are negatively affected. You may be avoiding work-related social events or conferences because of an attack or fear of having one. During a migraine episode, you may feel that your ability to interact with coworkers, your boss, or clients is impaired. A consequence of this is that you may feel that your job performance or job evaluation may be adversely affected.

There are steps, however, that you can take to minimize the risk of a migraine attack at work as well as ways to lower your level of stress. The first thing you should do is to identify triggers in your work environment. Questions 53 to 66 identify various environmental triggers. One common trigger in the work environment is poor lighting. Lighting should be bright enough for you to see clearly, but glaring or bright overhead fluorescent lighting can be a potential problem. You may want to use a desk lamp or floor lamp instead. You may also want to monitor the glare from the computer screen if you work at a computer, and be aware of your posture if you have a tendency to sit for long periods of time. Be aware of any tension in your upper back or neck, and be sure to take frequent rest and stretching breaks. Brief rest periods taken each hour can be extremely helpful in reducing muscle tension and overall emotional stress. Take a walk around the office, get a glass of water, or perhaps practice some simple breathing or relaxation techniques. You can sit at your desk or find a quiet place and practice some deep relaxing breaths for a few minutes. Question 94 describes some techniques that can be adapted to your work environment. You also can practice some easy stretching exercises to stretch your neck and shoulder muscles. The Feature at the end of this book illustrates easy-to-learn stretching exercises to reduce shoulder, neck, and scalp tension.

You should always be prepared with medication in case a migraine comes on while at work. Always have your medications with you, in your office, or at your work site. At the onset of a headache, take a break, try to relax, or find a quiet place to rest if possible. Be mindful of long meetings or conferences that may be a source of stress for you. Do what you can do to relax and practice the many techniques described in this book. Also, if missing a meal is a trigger for you, make sure you eat on time, and don't put off lunch or dinner because of work demands.

Finally, you can check with your employer or your human resources department to see what accommodations they can make to create a better work environment for you.

87. Should I tell my employer? What expectations can I have of my employer to accommodate my migraines?

The decision to inform your employer of your migraines is a personal choice that many migraine sufferers struggle with. If you feel your performance at essential job functions is being impaired by frequent attacks, you may want to speak with someone at your job about it. Often, migraineurs are worried that others will think they are just lazy, not competent, or hiding some medical or psychological problem. If this is the case, it might be appropriate to not only inform but also to educate your employer or colleagues about migraines and their consequences, specifically the impact on work performance.

Many employers are now well educated about migraines, and most are willing to make accommodations for employees with migraines. The Americans with Disabilities Act, passed by the U.S. Congress in 1990 and discussed in detail in Question 88, states that an employer must make "reasonable accommodations" for an employee with a disability. Reasonable accommodations provided by the employer may include allowing the employee to have a flexible or part-time work schedule, allowing a change in lighting or temperature if it does not impinge on other employees' work environment, or allowing rest periods or leave of absences if necessary.

However, because migraines are often thought of as an "invisible disorder," that is, a medical problem that can't be objectively "seen" by others, sometimes you may have to educate your employer about migraines. This may mean informing him or her that migraines are a legitimate neurological disorder. A report or letter from your doctor and written materials on migraines may be very useful. You and your employer will both likely be relieved after this is discussed. In the future, you may not feel shame about taking a day off or worry that you are perceived as less than an ambitious worker.

You may have to educate your employer about migraines.

Speaking to your employer can be difficult and stressful. If your supervisor is knowledgeable about migraines, you will have an easier time discussing it. When speaking to your employer, be direct and honest. Examine your reasons for wanting to speak with your boss. If you are dissatisfied with some aspect of your job, be careful not to use your headaches as a way of avoiding work. As stated, you may want to have a letter from your neurologist with you and make reading materials on migraines available if appropriate. Together, you can come to an agreement on what accommodations can be made to foster a better work environment. If the conversation doesn't go as well as you would have liked or if you feel he or she is not understanding or accommodating, check with your union, human resources department, or the U.S. Government website for the Americans with Disabilities Act at *http://www.ADA.gov*.

88. Can I be fired for poor work performance due to migraines? Is it possible to get disability for my headaches?

No, you can't be fired for having migraines. Migraines are a legitimate medical disorder, and migraine sufferers are protected by the Americans with Disabilities Act (ADA) passed by the United States Congress in 1990. The ADA prohibits discrimination "against a qualified individual with a disability." In order to be protected by the ADA, you must demonstrate that you are "disabled" *and* "qualified" to carry out your job functions either with or without a reasonable accommodation. The ADA defines a disability as a "physical or mental impairment that substantially limits one or more of the life activities of an individual; a record of such an impairment; or being regarded as having such an impairment."

As a migraineur, you may know from firsthand experience of the limitations an attack can place on you, including impairment in ability to communicate, think, concentrate, or perform effectively or even adequately. However, having migraines does not automatically allow an individual to be classified as a person with a disability. The severity of the migraine disorder and its impact on life activities is assessed, and if it is accepted that it meets the criteria for a disability, the employee still must be able to perform his or her job function with a reasonable accommodation by the employer. Migraines vary significantly in each person, and each work disability case is evaluated individually. Both the severity of the migraines and the potential accommodations for that employee by the employer are assessed. The two types of financial assistance available are the Supplemental Security Income (SSI) and Social Security Disability Insurance (SSDI), both of which fall under the authority of the Social Security Administration.

For more information on the Americans with Disabilities Act, you can contact the U.S. Department of Justice's official website at *http://www.ADA.gov*.

PART SIX

Complementary and Alternative Medicine

What is complementary and alternative medicine?

What are the primary treatments included in complementary and alternative medicine?

When should I consult with a CAM practitioner or think about using a complementary and alternative treatment?

More . . .

89. What is complementary and alternative medicine?

Complementary and alternative medicine, also commonly known as CAM, refers to a wide variety of healthcare practices and therapeutic approaches that fall outside the domain of conventional Western medicine. CAM focuses on the diagnosis, prevention, and treatment of disease through the application of a diverse assortment of practices. Increasingly over the years, patients have turned to complementary and alternative treatments seeking relief from an extensive variety of medical disorders including migraines. Complementary and alternative approaches are not intended to replace conventional medical treatment from your physician, but instead to serve in addition to it. The combination of complementary and alternative approaches and conventional medical treatment is commonly referred to as **integrative medicine**.

In addition to increased awareness of CAM by patients, there has been a growing body of scientific knowledge regarding the effectiveness of these treatments. In an effort to scientifically research and provide evidenced-based CAM treatments to the public, the U.S. Government's National Institutes of Health founded the National Center for Complementary and Alternative Medicine in 1998. Increasingly, medical doctors are referring patients to CAM practitioners, and medical schools are integrating nonconventional healthcare practices into their curriculums. Therapies and products that were once considered alternative or unconventional, such as biofeedback, acupuncture, and vitamins, are now part of mainstream healthcare practice.

Safety of Complementary and Alternative Therapies:

Despite the positive changes in the healthcare system, it is still easy for patients to feel confused when trying to assess the effectiveness of such a wide array of treatments and products. Alternative treatments range from approaches that have been scientifically researched and published in medical peer-reviewed journals to practices that can be extremely costly and have no proven therapeutic benefit. Some therapies or alternative remedies can even be harmful if combined with specific medications, contraindicated for your condition, or used in place of needed medical treatment. Chronic migraine sufferers are often desperate for effective treatments and might be eager to try approaches that promise relief. Always consult with your neurologist or physician treating your migraine when deciding to use a complementary medical approach. Complementary and alternative treatments, particularly the practices discussed in this chapter, can have significant potential for the prevention and treatment of migraine. This potential is optimized when used as a *supplement* to your medical treatment, or when you have received sufficient information that satisfies you on the safety and effectiveness of the treatment.

The following resources provide more information on complementary and alternative treatments:

- National Center for Complementary and Alternative Medicine/National Institutes of Health (*http://nccam.nih.gov*)
- White House Commission on Complementary and Alternative Medicine Policy (*http://www.whccamp.hhs.gov*)

90. What are the primary treatments included in complementary and alternative medicine?

Complementary and alternative treatments include a diverse and broad array of practices. CAM practices range from gentle, non-pharmacologic, and noninvasive treatments such as relaxation and breathing techniques to more invasive treatments such as chiropractic spinal manipulation, herbal medicine, and **acupuncture**.

The National Center for Complementary and Alternative Medicine of the National Institutes of Health classifies CAM treatments into the following five categories:

1. **Alternative Medical Systems:** These are alternate and comprehensive medical or healing systems, each with their own set of therapeutic techniques, practices, and belief systems. Some were founded within Western culture, such as **homeopathic medicine** and **naturopathic medicine**. Others were developed thousands of years ago in Eastern cultures such as traditional Chinese medicine and Ayurveda, which was developed in India. It is interesting to note that although these are considered alternative to conventional medical practice, many of these systems—particularly the Eastern medical systems—predate our present Western medical system by thousands of years.

2. **Mind–Body Interventions:** Mind–Body practices refer to a broad collection of approaches and therapies that have received considerable evidence-based support for their effectiveness in treating migraine, chronic pain, and other medical problems that may be exacerbated by emotional stress.

Acupuncture

A Chinese traditional therapy using fine needles inserted at specific points in the body to stimulate and regulate the flow of chi or vital energy to restore a healthy energy balance.

Homeopathic medicine

System of medicine based on concept of "like cures like"; symptoms are treated with minute doses of a substance that would normally produce the same symptoms as the illness being treated.

Naturopathic medicine

Healthcare system that uses diet, herbs, and other natural methods to treat illness.

Biofeedback

The use of electrical devices to recognize changes in body functions (heart rate, muscle tension) to achieve relaxation.

Mind–body techniques harness the mind's ability for natural healing and aim at using the innate wisdom of the mind to regulate emotional and bodily functions. These methods are believed to work by altering biological responses that are linked with stress and pain. Emotions and thoughts play a significant role in the course of *all* medical disorders. Since the experience of pain is frequently associated with a variety of emotional, psychological, and social factors, it is essential that skills aimed at reducing or alleviating stress be integrated into a migraine or headache pain treatment. Mind–body approaches are very effective at reducing the levels of anxiety, depression, sleep disturbance, and other negative reactions or psychological symptoms that are related to the chronic cycle of migraine episodes. These emotions or reactions can often prolong or intensify a migraine episode or predispose a person to a migraine attack. Mind–body approaches also help you learn how to regulate your own physical responses such as muscle tension that are often associated with migraines. Mind–body approaches are safe and widely accepted to be an important part of migraine and headache treatment. Examples of mind–body practices are **biofeedback, meditation**, relaxation, **breathing techniques, hypnosis, guided imagery, yoga**, and **creative visualization**.

3. **Biologic-Based Therapies:** Unlike noninvasive complementary and alternative approaches, this category of pharmacologic therapies is invasive and consists of using chemical substances, dietary supplements, and herbal products. While some

Meditation

Process of focused attention to cultivate increased awareness.

Breathing techniques

Variety of techniques that use patterned breathing to achieve relaxation.

Hypnosis

Range of techniques to foster a state of awareness where relaxation and self-suggestions are achieved.

Guided imagery

The use of mental images, visualization, and imagination to promote healing or changes in health, emotions, and behaviors.

Yoga

A discipline that promotes physical, emotional, and spiritual well-being through posture, stretches, breathing, and meditative exercises.

Creative visualization

The use of mental visual images to promote relaxation, healing, and changes in health and behavior.

Massage therapy

Pressure, massage, and manipulation of muscle and tissue in the treatment of musculoskeletal pain.

Rolfing

A deep form of manipulation of the muscles and fascia involved in musculoskeletal pain.

Chiropractic

The use of spinal manipulation to correct misalignments along the spine.

Osteopathy

School of medicine that provides comprehensive medical care with special attention to joints, bones, muscles, and nerves.

Shiatsu

Form of acupressure to maintain good health and relaxation.

Acupressure

A Chinese traditional therapy using finger pressure at specific points along the body.

Reiki

Traditional Chinese form of touch-based "energy healing."

Qi gong

Traditional Chinese energy therapy using movements, breathwork, and meditation.

of these substances, such as magnesium, the herbal remedy feverfew, and fish oil have received clinical evidence for the prevention or treatment of migraines (see Question 26), other treatments lack scientifically acceptable evidence regarding their effectiveness or safety. The risk of adverse effects in these practices is considerably higher than other CAM approaches, so caution should be used when using any product or "natural" substance without the approval of your physician.

4. **Body-Based Therapies:** Body-based therapies are a collection of noninvasive treatment practices based on the belief that many health problems can be prevented or treated through the manipulation or movement of body areas including soft tissue and the spine. In general, these are intended to complement conventional medical therapies and may aid in the prevention of migraines or in bringing quicker relief during an episode, particularly if neck, scalp, shoulder, and upper back muscle tension are present. Examples of body-based therapies are **massage therapy, Rolfing, chiropractic** and **osteopathy, Shiatsu, acupressure**, and cranial-sacral therapy.

5. **Energy Therapies:** This category of approaches is based on the concept of energy forces, either from the human body or through spiritual forces, which can be manipulated or "channeled" to facilitate a healing response. Many of these concepts are rooted in the foundations of ancient mystical healing practices. These approaches are increasingly popular, and although there are few adverse risks in the practices, the specific therapeutic effects have yet to be objectively measured. Examples include therapeutic touch, faith and spiritual healing, **Reiki, Qi gong**, and the application of magnets.

91. When should I consult with a CAM practitioner or think about using a complementary and alternative treatment?

At any time during the course of your migraine treatment, you may decide to consult with a practitioner of CAM. Seeking professional help for migraines is often an overwhelming and daunting task. Remember, this is *your* health and *your* team of healthcare professionals who are treating *your* migraine. Deciding when or how to find a medical doctor, CAM practitioner, or therapist is a highly individualized and personal choice. While a specific treatment may work for one migraineur, it may not provide any relief to another. Patients' responses to conventional and alternative treatments are highly individualized, and it is often through a system of trial and error that choices are reached regarding specific treatments. As with all therapies and professional healthcare providers that you may use (traditional or alternative), ultimately you will make the final decision as to your level of comfort with them.

People are increasingly using CAM for a diverse array of medical and psychological problems. According to the most recent study measuring the usage of CAM, 42% of the U.S. population has consulted with a practitioner of complementary and alternative medicine. People seek CAM for a variety of reasons. Occasionally they may find conventional treatments ineffective or the healthcare system too impersonal and institutionalized. Often they are seeking to use CAM in addition to their standard medical treatment. Your physician may recommend that you try alternative approaches in the prevention or treatment of your migraines, or you may come to that decision on your own. Either way, when thinking about using a complementary or alternative approach, it is first wise to consult with your physician.

92. *What considerations should I make when choosing a practitioner of CAM or when deciding to use an alternative approach?*

When considering an alternative approach for your migraine treatment, it is imperative that you first collect as much information as possible regarding the treatment you are seeking. This may come through consultations with your physician or other healthcare professionals or through acquiring information from the many written and online sources available. A good place to start is the National Institutes of Health's National Center for Complementary and Alternative Medicine (*http://nccam.nih.gov*), which provides detailed descriptions of alternative treatments and information on how to assess the quality of the online information you are receiving.

When contemplating using CAM, there are some important considerations that should be made regarding both the practitioner *and* the treatment approach. In reference to the practitioner, some questions to consider are:

- Does this person have a license or certificate in their respected field?
- What are the state regulations, qualifications, and standards for a person practicing this approach?
- What is the person's educational background?
- Does this person guarantee complete results and therefore sound unrealistic?
- Do I feel comfortable hiring this person to help in my treatment?

If you find you cannot receive adequate answers to these questions, you should proceed with caution and/or consult with another person. Most therapeutic approaches have detailed qualifications that a person must obtain to practice in that state. The Appendix lists professional organizations, licensing boards, and regulatory agencies for many complementary and alternative approaches.

When obtaining information regarding a specific therapy, questions that you should ask are:

- Is there evidence supporting this therapy for migraines?
- What is the quality of this evidence?
- Are results published in peer-reviewed and professional publications?
- Does my physician approve of this treatment?
- How safe is this treatment?
- What are the risks of this therapy?
- Is it invasive?
- Does it promise an instant cure for migraines or effective management? (Effective management is likely a more reasonable objective.)

Satisfactory answers to these questions should be obtained prior to beginning or continuing treatment.

Many of the approaches used in CAM are extremely safe and may play a very important role in the treatment of your migraines. It is usually unwise to presume that any single approach will cure or be the only therapy for your migraine. Always consult with your physician and use alternative practices as part of an integrated and effective treatment approach.

93. I often hear about the use of acupuncture. Is there evidence that acupuncture may help in the treatment of migraine?

Traditional Chinese medicine

System of medicine dating back thousands of years. Integrates a variety of ancient and modern therapies including acupuncture, herbal medicine, and massage to treat a wide range of medical conditions.

Acupuncture is a component of **traditional Chinese medicine** and was developed well over two thousand years ago. It is among the most studied and researched complementary and alternative therapies. As one of the most documented alternative therapies, it is widely accepted by conventional medicine as a treatment for a variety of pain conditions. Acupuncture treatment for migraine has received considerable clinical research attention in recent years and is currently widely applied as a treatment for headache and migraine pain.

Acupuncture is based on the belief that optimal health is achieved by maintaining a proper balance and flow of *chi* or *qi* (pronounced "chee"), the vital life force or energy. This energy is believed to move in the body through *meridians*, pathways that are each related to a specific organ. If this flow of *chi* becomes unbalanced either through excess or deficiency, pain and other bodily problems are believed to result. Acupuncture corrects this imbalance by inserting thin sterilized needles to appropriate points along the meridians to remove blockage and restore proper energy flow and balance. Needles are left in for roughly thirty minutes and cause little or no discomfort. A possible scientific explanation for its effectiveness in pain treatment is related to its stimulation and release of neurotransmitters known as endorphins, enkephalins, and serotonin. Endorphins and enkephalins are opioid peptides, the body's own personal painkilling chemicals. In addition to pain relief, there is strong evidence for the use of acupuncture in the treatment of nausea, and it therefore may be useful for nausea associated with migraines.

The scientific evidence on the effectiveness of acupuncture as a migraine treatment is promising, and studies support its role for prevention of migraine. Acupuncture appears to have success in reducing the frequency of migraine attacks. Acupuncture, when practiced by a qualified professional, is generally a safe treatment, and adverse effects are rare.

State regulations vary on the requirements to practice acupuncture. However, the majority of states require the practitioner to possess a licensure or certification in acupuncture. In addition, many MDs and DOs (Doctors of Osteopathy) now receive certification and/or licensure in acupuncture. You can check the requirements in your state by consulting the American Academy of Medical Acupuncture or the National Certification Commission for Acupuncture and Oriental Medicine, listed in the Appendix.

94. What are relaxation techniques, and are they helpful in my migraine treatment?

Before discussing the benefits of relaxation and the usefulness of relaxation techniques in the treatment of migraines, let us first briefly review a few things about stress and its impact on migraines. It is important to remember that stress does not initially *cause migraines*, but *does* trigger migraine attacks once you are vulnerable to them. As discussed in Question 60, stress mobilizes the "fight-or-flight" response that causes biochemical and vascular changes in the brain and also tightness or contractions in the muscles in your neck, shoulders, and scalp. These physical events can trigger a migraine attack in a person vulnerable to migraines. Stress is an unavoidable part of being alive. The goal of relaxation techniques is not to avoid stress in your life, but to help you avoid or minimize the harmful effects of stress on your health, and more specifically, to diminish the frequency and intensity of your migraine attacks.

Relaxation is an extremely important component of integrative migraine treatment. Some of the relaxation techniques described in this book include breathing exercises, meditation, progressive relaxation, biofeedback, guided imagery, and hypnosis. The one thing that all these various techniques have in common is that they help reduce the harmful effects of stress on the body. No one technique is necessarily better than any other; the important thing is that you practice some sort of technique to help self-regulate the biological effects of stress. You may want to try a few out and stick with the one that feels best. Each one, if practiced correctly, produces similar benefits. Learning relaxation techniques also gives you a sense of control over your health and migraines instead of feeling controlled by the consequences of frequent attacks.

Relaxation response

Physiological response associated with reduced stress and changes to heart rate, blood pressure, and breathing. The physiological and emotional opposite of the fight-or-flight response.

The Relaxation Response: Relaxation techniques are ways to bring about a deep state of relaxation or restfulness. This is not the same as sleep or simply lying down and "relaxing." These are techniques that when practiced correctly will leave you in a uniquely restful, but alert state of awareness. Herbert Benson, MD, of the Mind/Body Institute of Harvard Medical School has coined this state of relaxation the "relaxation response." The relaxation response is the common physiological response found in many types of relaxation, meditation, and spiritual prayer disciplines. Researchers have measured the biological responses of individuals in all types of relaxation and in many forms of prayer across many spiritual traditions and found this healing response to be elicited in each one.

The relaxation response is the psychological and physiological opposite of the "fight-or-flight" response discussed in Question 60. During the relaxation response, the sympathetic nervous system slows down. The sympathetic nervous system is part of the autonomic nervous system that plays a major role in migraines and stress, including regulating sleep, anxiety, and the size of blood vessels in the brain, all-important factors to the migraine sufferer. The effects of the relaxation response have extremely important implications for migraine sufferers. These effects include:

- A slowing down of heart rate
- Decrease in blood pressure
- Decrease in muscle tension
- Increase in oxygen utilization and improved oxygen flow to brain
- Increased blood flow
- Increase in more relaxed brain-wave rhythm
- Slowed and more efficient breathing rate
- Decrease in brain chemicals (catecholamines) that may stimulate migraines

General Guidelines on How to Elicit the Relaxation Response

There are two essential steps to eliciting the relaxation response:

1. Repetition of a word, sound, phrase, or spiritual word or phrase.
2. Passively disregarding everyday thoughts that inevitably come to mind, and returning to the repetition of the chosen word or phrase.

Here is one general, standard set of instructions used by Dr. Benson.[1] First, find a comfortable place to sit. This could be in a chair or sitting crossed-legged on the

[1] Adapted from *Timeless Healing, The Power and Biology of Belief* by Herbert Benson, MD, New York, NY: Scribner; 1996.

floor. If you use a chair, make sure it provides you with good support and that your back is fairly straight. It is wise not to lie down because you may fall asleep. Try to ensure that you will have 10 to 20 minutes of time with no distractions. Tell others in your household not to disturb you during this time. No telephones, no TV on in the background or other distractions. This is *your* quiet time. You can time yourself by occasionally glancing at a clock or watch.

1. Pick a focus word or short phrase that is firmly rooted in your personal belief system. This can simply be a neutral word like *one*, *peace*, or *love*. Alternatively, you can use a spiritual word or short phrase that you like.

2. Sit quietly in a comfortable position.

3. Close your eyes.

4. Relax your muscles.

5. Breathe slowly and naturally, repeating your focus word or phrase silently as you exhale.

6. Throughout, assume a passive attitude. Don't worry about how well you're doing. When other thoughts come to mind, simply and gently return to your repetition.

7. Continue for 10 to 20 minutes. You may open your eyes to check the time, but do not use an alarm. When you finish, sit quietly for a minute or so, at first with your eyes closed and later with your eyes open. Then, do not stand for one or two minutes.

8. Practice the techniques once or twice a day.

There are many ways to bring about a relaxed state and elicit the relaxation response. Other techniques or approaches that promote the effects of relaxation are described in the following paragraphs. Take your time in learning these various approaches. You may experience immediate benefits, but if you don't, do not despair. If one doesn't come easily, try another. Slowly incorporate one or more techniques into your daily routine. The cumulative effects on how your body reacts to stress will be well worth you staying with the practice. Often, you can be taught these techniques by CAM providers or clinical psychologists who specialize in health psychology or behavioral health. These techniques are also described in countless books, at community centers, and other health-related resources. Always check the qualifications of the source you are learning from. A list of resources can be found in the Appendix.

Breathing Techniques: You may think that breathing comes natural to you. You know how to breathe. You do it all the time! Well, although this is true, it is rare that we give the breath the amount of attention it deserves. Many health experts now agree that attending to our breathing process may be one of the most powerful self-healing techniques we can perform. For thousands of years, breathing techniques have been at the core of many approaches to promote optimal physical and mental health. Even though you are constantly breathing, chances are you are not paying attention to the breathing process. When under stress or in pain, people usually switch to a breathing style that might only promote additional stress, anxiety, and more pain. When done correctly, breath work is a powerful tool to decrease stress, anxiety, and pain.

An individual who is having a migraine or is under severe stress is likely to be breathing with shallow breaths, primarily from the chest or thoracic area. This type of breathing is associated with panic, anxiety, and pain. Proper breathing, as discussed in the section on the relaxation response, evokes the opposite of the "fight-or-flight" response, which is associated with stress. Effective relaxation techniques can alter and lower levels of specific neurotransmitters in the brain that are associated with stress and headaches when they are at high levels. One effective way to breathe correctly is what is called **diaphragmatic breathing**.

Diaphragmatic breathing

A method of breathing in which the breath originates in the abdomen rather than the chest. This method is thought to allow for more effective relaxation.

Diaphragmatic breathing is a breathing style where the breath originates from the diaphragm or belly instead of the chest area. To begin with, ideally you should be in a calm and restful place and mood (although with a little practice relaxation breathing can certainly be practiced anywhere). Assume a comfortable sitting or lying down position and begin by inhaling gently through your nose. Breathing through the nose results in a more direct and purified air stream to the brain. While you inhale through your nose, be aware of the breath filling up your abdomen while it gently expands. Your abdomen should be expanding with each inhalation and contracting with each exhalation. You can feel this by resting your hand on your belly. If your shoulders and chest are rising with each breath, then you are breathing from your chest and not breathing deeply into the abdomen. Try to leave your chest and shoulders still while your belly fills up with air.

Continue with this process for a few minutes by breathing into your abdomen while it expands and then exhaling through your slightly open mouth. This may at first seem a little difficult and unnatural to do, but soon you will become very familiar with this breathing. Indeed, in a short time, this will seem a natural way to breathe. In fact, if you ever watch an infant breathing, the baby breathes from the abdomen; you can watch the belly expanding with each inhalation. Once you are comfortable with this style of breathing, you can practice this anytime you choose, especially at times of high stress or at the onset of a headache.

You can also combine diaphragmatic breathing with deep breathing. Take long, slow deep breaths through your nose and exhale through your mouth using your abdomen. Just a few minutes of this can result in a more physically and emotionally restful but alert state.

Guided Imagery: Guided imagery, also known as creative visualization, is a pleasant way to both relax and, with the use of your imagination, promote a healing emotional and bodily response. Guided imagery and visualization are relaxation techniques where you use your imagination to create fantasies or scenes where you picture yourself relaxed, peaceful, unstressed, and without migraines. You might picture yourself in a tranquil setting such as a beach or mountain lake with your body and mind at total ease. This may be combined with breathing techniques to help bring on a relaxed state. In addition to visualizing peaceful settings to relax mind and body, you may picture physical changes occurring that would alleviate a migraine, such as picturing blood vessels or muscles that may be inflamed during an attack slowly constricting. This technique is very similar to **clinical hypnosis**. There is a lot of room for creativity here. For instance, you may picture the pain in your head as red in color, and then slowly with your imagination (or with the aid of a skilled therapist) change the color to blue or green or any color that

Clinical hypnosis

Range of techniques to foster a state of awareness where relaxation and self-suggestions are achieved to bring about behavioral and emotional changes. Used commonly in pain, headaches, phobias, and anxiety.

invokes a more comfortable and cooler feeling. If you have an active imagination and enjoy this type of activity, this may be very helpful for you. Scientific evidence has found that creative visualization and guided imagery can have a positive impact on bodily functions, promote healing, and reduce sickness.

There are many books, audiotapes, and CDs that can be helpful. Many psychologists and other licensed mental health professionals practice guided imagery or visualization. Resources and recommended readings on guided imagery/visualization are listed in the Appendix.

Clinical Hypnosis: Also known as hypnotherapy or self-hypnosis, this is a relaxed and focused state of awareness. In many ways, it is similar to guided imagery and creative visualization. Working with a qualified hypnotherapist, in your imagination you will enter into a relaxed, restful state whereby you will be open to verbal suggestions, images, and visualizations that will help you relax and directly alleviate or prevent migraines. It may feel like you are daydreaming. Actually, when you are daydreaming you are in a similar trance-like state of awareness.

Many people have misconceptions about hypnosis, most likely because they have seen hypnotists perform as part of some entertainment show where they seem to cause people to do things against their will and without knowing it. *This is simply not true and is not what a qualified healthcare provider who practices clinical hypnosis does.* You are in complete control at all times and alert to your surroundings. Clinical hypnosis is just a method to bring you into a state of focused concentration where you can use the power of the mind–body connection to promote a healing response. An example of how it might be used in migraine pain is that after being brought into a deep and relaxed trance, you might be given suggestions to lower your pain. This may include being asked to lower an imaginary dial that controls pain in your head or to imagine the pain leaving your head as you imagine your blood vessels returning to their normal size. It can be used also to help with anxiety, fear, and other difficult and challenging emotions. After you have done this with a qualified therapist for a brief number of sessions, you can then learn to recreate this experience on your own. This is often referred to as self-hypnosis. Scientific evidence supports its use in managing pain.

Because no licensure is required to specifically practice hypnosis, it is recommended that you choose a licensed mental health professional such as a clinical psychologist, psychiatrist, or clinical social worker, or choose a therapist credentialed from a reputable professional hypnosis organization. You may contact the organizations listed in the Appendix for more information on hypnosis and on how to find a practitioner.

95. I've been told that learning meditation may be helpful. Exactly what is meditation, and is it helpful in treating migraines and stress?

Undoubtedly you have heard of meditation, and perhaps you have even learned various meditative techniques. We want to review the importance of learning to meditate as an effective way of working with the emotional and physical symptoms associated with migraines. Often people think of meditation as some mystical practice whereby they are to somehow empty the mind of all thoughts. Or else people say to themselves, "I could never meditate" or "I don't have the spiritual training to do that." These are some of the many misconceptions regarding meditation. Although meditation dates to ancient times and early religious practices, it can be practiced without any religious or philosophical context, and is gaining an increasing amount of attention as a therapeutic treatment.

A growing amount of research is now documenting the benefits of meditation on conditions such as headaches, chronic pain, immune disorders, depression, anxiety, stress, heart disease, and cancer. In recent years, meditation has become popular both in the popular culture and also in healthcare settings as a very effective method to evoke physical and emotional states of relaxation, and also to learn an effective way of paying attention to both the mind and body. In doing this, meditation is highly useful in learning to self-regulate the emotional and physical activity that is often associated with migraines as well as daily life stress. Once incorporated as part of a daily routine, meditation has the potential to provide you with benefits to mind and body that can be both enjoyable and enduring.

Meditation may be generally understood as a way of paying attention to one's self (body and mind) in the present moment. It is also a method that promotes a physical and emotional state of relaxation that results in the benefits described in Question 94. However, in addition to the wide range of benefits to general health and to the reduction of symptoms linked with many illnesses, meditation is unique in that it introduces a useful way to increase awareness of our emotional and physical processes. Meditation creates a state of relaxation and alert attention whereby you observe all things happening in the present moment just as they are. These include the many thoughts running through your mind, the sensations in your body, or the emotions you may be feeling. One misconception is that meditation is cultivating an empty mind. Actually, meditation is learning to mindfully cultivate an awareness of what is happening in your body and mind in the present moment. By attending to these mind and body events in the following ways, you can gain a new perspective on how you emotionally and physically react to stress. It is also an excellent method for altering your perception of pain. Meditation is the art of focused attention. By paying attention to the present moment, you can enjoy a wide range of health benefits as you develop an emotionally stable, calm, and nonreactive response to stressful events.

Meditation usually involves focusing the attention on a single object such as the breath, an image, or a sound, word, or phrase, also known as a *mantra*. While you focus your attention on an object such as a word or breath, you will notice that your mind eventually drifts to arising thoughts, emotions, or bodily sensations. When you become aware that your attention has shifted to any thought, emotion, or physical sensation other than your object of focus, gently bring your attention back to the object of focus. This is done without self-judgment. Just simply acknowledge that you have drifted to thinking about work, perhaps to a feeling regarding a family member, or maybe to some discomfort in your body. Gently repeat this process of focusing attention and returning to your breath (or chosen word) over and over as your attention wanders. This process of the mind wandering and returning to the object of focus is the process of meditation.

Mindfulness meditation, also known as insight meditation, cultivates moment-to-moment awareness of the thoughts, emotions, and physical sensations that are constantly rising and falling in your consciousness. The meditator is taught to be aware of all thoughts, feelings, perceptions, images, smells, sounds, and sensations that occur constantly in the mind without becoming attached, involved, or reactive to any one item in particular. As thoughts, feelings, and sensations come and go, you are not to ignore or suppress them or, conversely, to judge or investigate them. When your mind drifts to a thought, feeling, or bodily sensation, you just make a mental note of where your mind is and return to the breath and the process of observing all things as they occur in the present moment. This process of increasing awareness of emotions, thoughts, and physical sensations as they occur will over time become easier for you and allow you to be less reactive to stressful events as they occur in daily life. Dr. Jon Kabat-Zinn, who has written an excellent and highly recommended book titled *Full Catastrophe Living* has stated that it is this ". . . discerning observation of whatever comes up in the present moment that is the hallmark of mindfulness and differentiates it most from other forms of meditation. The goal of mindfulness is for you to be more aware, more in touch with life and whatever is happening in your body and mind at the time it is happening . . . that is, the present moment."

Meditation has been taught to thousands of migraine and headache sufferers with very positive results all over the nation and at many medical centers and hospitals. For more information on mindfulness meditation, please consult the resources in the Appendix under *Meditation*.

96. What is biofeedback, and how helpful is it in migraine treatment?

Biofeedback is one of the most popular and researched mind–body techniques used in the treatment of migraine headaches. Biofeedback training is a safe and valuable technique used to help people learn to regulate physical symptoms that worsen many medical problems, including migraines. Biofeedback training uses different relaxation techniques (e.g., meditation, guided imagery, and progressive relaxation) combined with the use of instruments that measure various bodily functions. This helps a person learn to control physiological functions such as muscle tension, blood pressure, skin temperature, heart rate, and rate of breathing.

As discussed in Question 94, the state of relaxation evokes a unique biological response that is the physical opposite of the stress response (i.e., fight-or-flight response) that often accompanies or triggers a migraine episode. To get *feedback* on these biological changes, the instruments monitor information on the physical changes that occur during the relaxation process, such as heart rate, muscle tension, and breathing. In a typical biofeedback session, electrodes are placed on the patient's skin (a harmless process), which are connected to a computer that monitors the moment-to-moment physical changes as they occur. Through visual or auditory signals, you receive feedback on the physical changes you are producing.

One of the most popular types of feedback in migraine treatment is **electromyographic (EMG) biofeedback**, which measures muscle tension. Because migraine headaches are often accompanied or triggered by severe muscle tension in the upper back, neck, or scalp, learning

Electromyographic (EMG) biofeedback

Technique that uses sensors attached to muscles that are tense during migraines to attain muscle relaxation.

to reduce muscle tension can help in the prevention or decrease of the severity of a migraine episode. In EMG biofeedback, sensors are attached to problem body areas that are often tense for you. With the assistance of a qualified therapist, you will be given suggestions on how to feel more relaxed through mind–body techniques such as guided imagery, breathing techniques, or meditation. As the muscle tension in your scalp, forehead, neck, or upper back decreases, you will receive instant feedback via the monitors, thus increasing your awareness of how relaxation directly produces changes in muscle tension. It is not required that you receive feedback to experience the objectives of relaxation.

Another kind of biofeedback used in the treatment of migraines is thermal biofeedback. In this approach, hand sensors are attached to monitor the temperature of your hands. You are then given instructions on how to warm your hands, using your mind and breath. It is believed that by warming and raising the temperature of your hands, you are redirecting blood flow from your head. Vascular changes resulting from blood flow to the head are believed to play a part in migraine episodes. Biofeedback also can simply measure and give you feedback on the breath rate. By learning to bring about a general state of relaxation through proper changes in breathing, you can quickly discover the connection between effective breathing techniques and relaxation.

Biofeedback is safe and has no side effects. With the aid of a skilled and qualified therapist, you can learn how to control important bodily processes that can result in overall improved emotional and physical health. Once you have gained greater awareness on how to regulate or control bodily functions that are associated with your migraines, you can proceed with these techniques without the instruments used in biofeedback at any time on your own. This can be done regularly as a preventive measure against migraines or can be done at the first sign of an attack in an attempt to shorten the duration or lessen the severity of the migraine episode.

Many, but not all biofeedback therapists are clinical psychologists. Minimal requirements should be a license to practice psychology in your state and a certificate in biofeedback training. As with any therapist you consult with, you must feel comfortable and believe this expert is qualified to help you. Make sure the therapist is familiar with migraines and has had success in treating migraine patients. The Appendix resources listed under *Biofeedback* may be helpful in locating a biofeedback therapist near you.

97. How do massage and other body-based therapies prevent or treat migraine?

Massage therapy and other body-based therapies are excellent and often underutilized therapeutic approaches in the treatment of headaches and other chronic pain conditions. We frequently refer patients with chronic migraine or tension headaches for massage therapy. Therapeutic massage and other body-based therapies are effective in many significant ways. To begin with, massage produces a wonderful feeling of relaxation. Taking time out to relax in a tranquil setting and experience a massage is a great way to take care of and nurture yourself. Massage can reduce overall physical and emotional stress, improve mental clarity, increase lymphatic circulation, enhance energy, and improve sleep. There is growing scientific evidence that therapeutic massage may lower the levels of neurochemicals in the brain that are linked with stress and anxiety.

An important benefit and one directly related to the physical mechanism of migraines is that therapeutic massage directly relaxes the muscle tension in your upper back, neck, scalp, and face. Migraineurs frequently suffer from musculoskeletal constriction or tension, muscle spasms, and severe tightness or rigidity of the fascia, a broad band of connective tissue that surrounds muscles and organs. The fascia and muscles in the neck and head region may become extremely constricted during a migraine attack. This can produce significant pain and discomfort. Severe myofascial (muscle and fascia) pain can also trigger a migraine or tension headache episode. Often, people with migraines and tension headaches experience chronic tension in the muscles or fascia in the upper back, neck, and head, whereby a physical or emotional trigger can further increase these contractions and thus cause a full-blown migraine or tension headache. Upper back and neck muscles that are chronically contracted are also likely to have less oxygen flowing through those areas. Soft tissue pain can also result from trigger points, very hard and intense knots of muscular tension that can radiate pain to other parts of the body. You may sometimes feel these hard little knots in your neck muscles during a migraine or when you experience severe muscle tightness. These trigger points, like myofascial tightness, can produce intense pain, often adding to the pain you may already be feeling from the migraine.

Massage therapy, particularly massage that works at the deeper muscle layers, fascia, and trigger points, can bring about significant relief. For the greatest benefit and as a preventive measure against a build-up of muscle tightness or stress, you can choose to have massage treatments on a regular basis. You may find that this reduces the frequency of your migraines. Another effective strategy that may work for you is to have a massage before stressful events, weekends (if you suffer from weekend or "letdown" migraines), or before travel or a planned vacation. Thinking ahead and trying to pre-empt an episode is an effective coping strategy!

Always consult with your physician prior to starting any deep tissue massage treatment. Deep tissue massage is not for everyone, as there are some medical problems, including high blood pressure, serious infections, cancer, or circulatory problems, that could be exacerbated with intense pressure to the body.

There are many schools of massage therapy. Many differ in their underlying philosophy or the techniques used. When integrated into your migraine treatment, you may find these body-based therapies offer stress reduction, decrease the frequency and shorten the duration of your migraines, alleviate physical migraine triggers, and contribute to a general state of improved health. If one approach doesn't work, feel free to try a different approach or consult with another therapist. The following are the most common and widely used types of massage therapies:

Deep Tissue Massage: Deep tissue massage is a common technique and is often very effective in migraine, headache, and myofascial disorders of the neck and head. Deep tissue massage is performed with firm, moderate pressure and stretching to release chronic muscular tension. A therapist treating your migraine or headache can work deeply in the upper back, neck, and scalp areas, providing myofascial release and relief from headache pain. You should always feel comfortable to communicate to your therapist if the pressure is too much for you.

Neuromuscular massage

Technique that works by applying deep pressure to trigger points, a common cause of muscle pain in headache and myofascial disorders.

Neuromuscular Massage and **Trigger Point Work:** These techniques both work by applying deep pressure to trigger points, a common cause of muscle pain in headache and myofascial disorders as well as chronic pain conditions such as fibromyalgia. Pressure is applied with fingers or elbows until these knots of muscle tension soften and break up, resulting in greater circulation of blood flow and pain relief.

Acupressure and **Shiatsu:** Acupressure and Shiatsu are both based on the principles of Chinese medicine and acupuncture (Question 93) and are performed by applying finger pressure to specific points to promote a proper flow of energy (*chi*) and release blockages. It is very commonly used in headache disorders, including migraines, by applying pressure to specific points on the head promoting circulation and reducing muscle tension. You can experiment yourself by applying pressure to various points along your scalp and head. If you find relief at any point, you can self-apply pressure at any time. There are many books that show various acupressure points for pain and headache relief.

Rolfing: This is the most aggressive of the massage therapies and is clearly not for those people who don't like aggressive bodywork. Rolfing is based on the principle that pain and body dysfunction are caused by poor body alignment. Rolfing attempts to bring the body back in proper structural balance by applying very deep pressure and manipulation to the fascia, the deep connective tissue surrounding bones and organs in the body. Rolfing is the deepest of all bodywork treatments and can at times be very uncomfortable. However, it can be effective and is best indicated for those migraineurs with very severe muscle and myofascial constriction in the neck, head, and other parts of the body.

Swedish Massage: Swedish massage is probably the most well known type of massage therapy. It does not work as deeply as the other approaches mentioned and may not provide the proper pressure to bring myofascial or trigger point relief, however, it is a very relaxing and soothing treatment that can induce a state of relaxation and be the perfect therapy for you to help reduce stress. You may choose to have a Swedish massage after a migraine episode to help calm your body and mind down. Swedish massage is done with broad soothing strokes to the body and may also include kneading and movement of various muscle groups.

Swedish massage

Form of massage involving long strokes and kneading of muscle. Treats muscle tension and promotes overall relaxation.

There are many places to find a qualified massage therapist or other bodywork practitioner. Therapists often work in private practice settings, pain or rehabilitation centers, wellness centers, health clinics, or at well-known health spas. States vary as to the regulations required to practice. Many states now require a license to practice any type of massage or bodywork in addition to certification for the particular technique practiced. Always ensure that the minimal requirements are met, usually a state license and certification in the specific specialty you are seeking. The following professional organizations can provide you with the requirements of your state and list practitioners who are certified in their respective specialty (full listings for each organization are in the Appendix):

- American Massage Therapy Association
- National Certification Board for Therapeutic Massage and Bodywork
- The Rolf Institute

98. Are there specific stretching exercises I can do for my shoulder, neck, and head pain?

A common complaint of migraine and tension headache sufferers is that of chronic muscle tension in the upper back, neck, and scalp. This in itself can be quite painful and is often associated with the onset of tension headaches and may even assist in triggering a migraine episode. Tension headaches are often experienced concurrently with migraines for many patients. One theory is that tension and migraine headaches fall along a continuum and that muscle tension is part of most migraines.

One important method of reducing muscle tension and preventing chronic muscle tension build-up is stretching the muscles and soft tissue involved. Stretching is often underappreciated as a vital exercise in maintaining a healthy, flexible, and functional body. By practicing a few stretching exercises a day you can help prevent build up of chronic musculoskeletal or myofascial tension, and can even effectively reduce pain and discomfort during an acute episode. This can help reduce the intensity and potentially stop a tension headache from continuing. A collection of stretching exercises that may be helpful is presented in the Feature at the end of this book.

99. How do I find a complementary and alternative practitioner?

After deciding that one or more of the complimentary or alternative approaches discussed in this section may be right for your migraine treatment and you have reviewed the considerations (Question 92) in choosing a CAM provider, the next step is finding a practitioner. Just as selecting an alternative therapy may seem at first a daunting task, locating a qualified practitioner near you may also seem at first a little overwhelming. There are thousands of practitioners to choose from, and you are undoubtedly bombarded with advertisements for various clinicians promising migraine headache relief. As mentioned earlier, it is essential that you take responsibility for putting together your migraine treatment team.

One place to start when searching for a CAM practitioner is with your primary medical doctor or neurologist treating your migraines. If you are in treatment with a mental health professional such as a clinical psychologist, psychiatrist, or clinical social worker, they also may be very helpful in helping you locate a qualified practitioner for the therapy you have decided to pursue. A medical doctor who practices *integrative medicine* will likely know of qualified alternative medicine professionals.

A headache clinic or pain center is also an excellent place to locate a host of healthcare providers who treat migraine headaches and other pain conditions. There are many free-standing centers as well as hospital-based pain centers that are affiliated with a medical school. Most have a multidisciplinary team that consists of pain specialists including medical doctors, psychologists, psychiatrists, nurses, and CAM providers. If they don't have the type of therapist you are seeking, chances are good that they can provide you with some suggestions.

Finally, you can consult the Appendix, which lists national and regional organizations as well as professional membership organizations and societies. Many of these resources will provide you with a list of qualified, licensed, or credentialed alternative healthcare providers in your area.

100. Where can I get more information about migraines?

One book cannot answer all the questions you may have or address all the factors involved in migraines. The Appendix that follows contains organizations, websites, books, and other sources of information that may prove useful to you. You will also find a number of resources, reprinted here courtesy of the American Academy of Neurology, that may be helpful to you and your physician as you document your migraines, their triggers, and any associated events.

Exercises for Migraine Prevention

DISCLAIMER

Be sure to consult your physician before undertaking any exercise program.

Introduction

Upper body postural distortion that has been linked to cervicogenic and migraine headaches is known as **upper crossed syndrome**. It is characterized by forward-thrust head, rounded shoulders and back, internally rotated arms, and a sunken chest. The exercises described on the following pages serve to counteract this posture and move the musculoskeletal system back into a healthier, more functional position.

First, the shortened muscles (underarm—latissimus dorsi; chest—pectoralis major/minor; neck—upper trapezius, levator scapulae, scalenes, and sternocleidomastoid) are stretched or released. This stretching lessens their dominance in this dysfunctional muscular pattern. Next, the opposing muscles that are lengthened and weak (stabilizers of the scapula: rhomboids; muscles in the mid-back between shoulder blades—serratus anterior, middle and lower trapezius) are activated, first in isolation and then in coordination with the entire system. This reinforces the flexibility of the muscles that were just stretched and stabilizes the newly created mobility. The goal of this program is to create new patterns of muscle movement that will improve the functioning and health of the neck and back.

For maximum results, in addition to performing this exercise routine on a daily basis, active awareness of your posture is the key to lasting improvements. There are other helpful maneuvers that may be practiced throughout the day. Take advantage of walls—they are great for postural alignment. Stand up against the wall whenever and wherever the opportunity presents itself. While standing against the wall draw your abdominals in toward your spine and pull your shoulder blades back and together. Perform these simple actions as often as possible and soon you will feel and look taller.

Exercise #1   Scalene Stretch

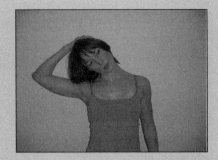

Stand up against a wall, tuck your chin inward and slowly draw your right ear toward your right shoulder. Your right hand can be used to apply slight pressure to assist this action. Hold stretch for 20 seconds and repeat on the opposite side. Complete two sets.

Reason: This exercise stretches the scalene muscles, which extend from your second through seventh cervical vertebrae down the side of your neck to your first two ribs. Lengthening these muscles increases the mobility of your shoulders, head, and upper spine.

Exercise #2   Levator Scapulae Stretch

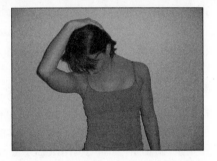

Stand up against a wall and tuck your chin inward, make a three quarter turn with your head, and draw your chin to your chest. Your right hand can be used to apply slight pressure to assist in this stretch. Hold stretch for 20 seconds and repeat on opposite side. Complete two sets.

Reason: This exercise stretches the levator scapulae muscle, which extends from your top four cervical vertebrae down the back of your neck to the top of your scapula. Lengthening this muscle increases the mobility of your shoulders, head, and upper spine.

Exercise #3   Sternocleidomastoid
Stretch

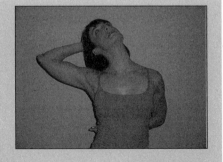

Place your right hand behind your back, squeeze your shoulder blades back and together, make a three quarter turn to the right with your head, and lift your chin to the ceiling. Your left hand may be used to apply slight pressure to assist in this stretch. Hold stretch for 20 seconds and repeat on opposite side. Complete two sets.

Reason: This exercise stretches the sternocleidomastoid muscle, which extends from the top of your sternum to the mastoid process behind your ear. Lengthening this muscle increases the mobility of your shoulders, head, and upper spine.

Exercise #4   Doorway Chest Stretch

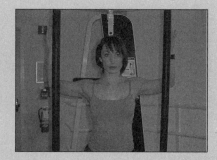

Stand in a doorway with your elbows bent at a 90 degree angle, draw your abdominals in toward your spine, and slowly allow your torso to fall forward until you feel a slight stretch through your chest and shoulders. Hold stretch for 20 seconds. Repeat one time.

Reason: This exercise stretches the pectoralis major and minor, which extend across your chest from the sides of your sternum (chest bone) to the top of your humerus (upper arm bone). Lengthening this muscle increases the mobility of the shoulder and upper spine.

Exercise #5   Single Arm Latissimus Dorsi Stretch

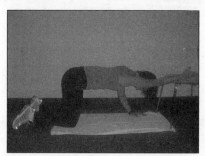

Begin by kneeling in front of a chair. Place your hand and forearm on the chair with your palm facing the ceiling. Draw your abdominals in toward your spine and move your knees back until your torso is parallel to the floor and you feel a stretch under your arm. Maintain your abdominal engagement and try to keep your spine in a neutral position (try not to arch your back) throughout the duration of the stretch. Hold for 30 seconds on both sides. Repeat one time.

Reason: This exercise stretches the latissimus dorsi muscle, which extends across the back from the lower thoracic and lumbar vertebrae, lower three to four ribs and iliac crest (top of pelvis) to the humerus (upper arm bone). Lengthening these muscles increases the mobility of the shoulder and increases the stability of both the pelvis and the shoulder.

Exercise #6   Upper Spinal Floor Twist

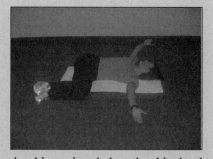

Lie on your side, bending your knees up at a 90 degree angle to your hips. Your arms are stretched out directly in front of your shoulders. Your head is resting on the floor or on a small flat pillow if you do not have the mobility to rest it on the floor. Slowly open your arms by reaching your top arm to the other side of your body. Your palm should stay facing the ceiling and your arm should not drop below shoulder level. Your knees should remain stacked on top of one another the entire time. DO NOT LET THEM SLIDE APART. Hold for one minute on both sides.

Reason: This exercise stretches the pectoral muscles, internal rotators of the shoulders, anterior deltoid, obliques and rectus abdominus, erector spinae muscles that run along the side of your spine, scalenes, and sternocleidomastoid neck muscles. Lengthening these muscles increases mobility of the thoracic and lumbar spine and shoulder complex, and creates a greater range of motion at the shoulder joint and in rotation of the torso.

Exercise #7   Chair-Assisted Back Release

Lie on your back with your knees bent at a 90 degree angle over a chair. Spread arms out at a 45 degree angle with your palms facing the ceiling. Relax into this position and notice if your back is evenly flattening onto the floor on both sides. Hold for five to ten minutes.

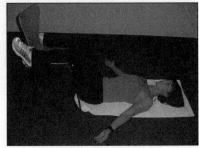

Reason: This exercise helps to release the paraspinal muscles (the muscles along the sides of the spine), realign the spine, and stabilize the pelvis.

Exercise #8   Chair-Assisted Back Release with Shoulder Contraction

Lie in the chair-assisted back release position with arms directly out to the side, elbows bent at a 90 degree angle with fisted hands, knuckles facing the ceiling. Draw your abdominals into your spine and squeeze your shoulder blades back and together and then release. Try to do this action without tensing your neck muscles. Do 30 repetitions.

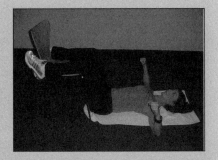

Reason: This exercise activates the rhomboids, lower trapezius, rear deltoids, and abdominals. It promotes extension through your upper back or thoracic spine.

Exercise #9   Shoulder Contractions

Stand up against a wall with your head, heels, pelvis, shoulders, and head touching the wall. Draw your abdominals in toward your spine, and pull your shoulder blades back and together and then release. Try to do this action without tensing your neck muscles. Do 30 repetitions.

Reason: This exercise activates the lower trapezius, rhomboids, and rear deltoids (the muscles in your upper back). Stengthening these muscles promotes mobility of the scapulae and thoracic (upper) spine. It promotes shoulder and spinal stability.

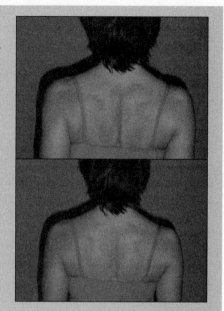

Exercise #10   Elbow Touches against Wall, Inward & Outward

Stand up against a wall with your head, heels, pelvis, shoulders, and head touching the wall. Draw your abdominals in toward your spine, make fists with your hands and place your knuckles on your temples. Your thumbs should point down toward the floor. Draw your elbows in toward each other, keeping your back against the wall, and then open your elbows by pulling them back toward the wall. Try to touch the wall with your elbows, but only pull them back as far as you can without losing your abdominal engagement or your contact with the wall. Try to do this action without tensing your neck muscles. If your neck muscles are dominating the exercise and it is difficult to release them, you may do this exercise with your hands placed on the tops of your shoulders. Do 30 repetitions.

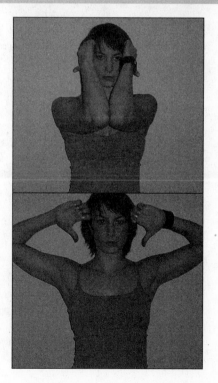

Reason: This exercise activates the abdominals, pectoral muscles, anterior and medial deltoids, serratus anterior (chest and shoulder muscles) while moving into the forward position. It activates the lower trapezius, rhomboids, and rear deltoids (upper back and rear shoulder muscles) while moving into the back position. Strengthening and stretching these muscles reciprocally promotes mobility of the shoulder and thoracic spine. These actions and the positioning up against the wall promote stability of the shoulder, spine, pelvis, knee, and ankle joints.

Exercise #11   Wall Squat with Arms at 90 Degree Angles

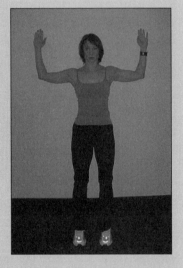

Stand with your back and head against a wall, move your feet about two feet away from the wall, making sure that they are hip width apart and parallel to each other with both toes facing forward. Draw your abdominals into your spine pressing your low back into the wall. Stretch your arms directly out to the side of your body with your palms facing outward. Try keeping your hands at shoulder level. Bend your knees, sliding your pelvis down the wall as if you were sitting in a chair. Make sure that your kneecaps are facing forward and positioned over your heels. Only go down as far as you can without losing the contact between your lower back and the wall. If your neck muscles begin to engage (tense up), stop here and lower your arms to a 45 degree verses 90 degree angle from your torso. If you are able to keep your neck released, continue by bending your elbows at a 90 degree angle and attempting to place the backs of your hands against the wall. Try to do this action without tensing your neck muscles. If you are unable to keep your neck relaxed, go back to the straight arm position either at shoulder level or lower. You may feel a stretch across your chest into your arms and the activation (characteristic of a muscle burn) of the muscles across your back and in your thighs. Hold this position for 30 seconds to start, and slowly increase your time to 2 minutes as you get stronger.

Reason: This exercise activates the abdominals, quadriceps, external rotators of the arm, extensors of the spine and head, hip flexors, and knee flexors isometrically. Strengthening these muscles promotes mobility and stability of the spine, pelvis and the shoulder, knee, and ankle joints. It is a total body exercise that incorporates all of the progress that was made in the previous exercises and helps to formulate a new, healthier muscular pattern.

Lara Licharowicz is the master trainer for the Advantage program and a Flexibility Specialist for the Sports Club LA in New York City. She has worked for the Sports Club LA at their 61st St. location, where she has been one of their most popular trainers, for four years. In addition, she has her own business and trains clients in the privacy of their own homes. Before becoming a personal trainer, Lara danced professionally for seven years touring throughout the United States, Asia, and Europe. Through learning and performing the work of several different choreographers, she developed her kinesthetic eye. She graduated with honors from SUNY-Purchase with a BFA in dance and a minor in psychology. She holds certifications in different aspects of personal training from the American Council on Exercise, National Academy of Sports Medicine, Maternal Fitness (Pre-Post Natal Training) and Power Pilates (Mat Training). She has also studied Functional Fitness with Juan Carlos Santana and is currently finishing work on her certification from the Egoscue Clinic, which is a method for non-medical pain relief. She strives daily to give her clients the best training the industry has to offer and is proud of her clients' success stories.

Organizations and Resources

Headaches and Pain Management

American Academy of Neurology
1080 Montreal Avenue
St. Paul, MN 55116
Tel: (800) 879-1960
Fax: (651) 695-2791
http://www.aan.com
email: memberservices@aan.com

American Academy of Pain Management
13947 Mono Way, #A
Sonora, CA 95370
Tel: (209) 533-9744
Fax: (209) 533-9750
http://www.aapainmanage.org

American Council for Headache Education (ACHE)
19 Mantua Road
Mount Royal, NJ 08061
Tel: (856) 423-0258
Fax: (856) 423-0082
http://www.achenet.org

American Headache Society
19 Mantua Road
Mount Royal, NJ 08061
Tel: (856) 423-0043
Fax: (856) 423-0082
http://www.americanheadachesociety.org

American Medical Association
515 North State Street
Chicago, IL 60610
Tel: (800) 621-8335
Fax: (312) 464-4184
http://www.ama-assn.org

American Pain Foundation
201 N. Charles Street, Suite 710
Baltimore, MD 21201-4111
Tel: (888) 615-PAIN (7246)
http://www.painfoundation.org

American Pain Society
4700 W. Lake Avenue
Glenview, IL 60025
Tel: (847) 375-4715
Fax: (847) 375-6480
http://www.ampainsoc.org

International Headache Society
http://www.i-h-s.org

**MAGNUM (Migraine Awareness Group:
A National Understanding for Migraineurs)**
100 North Union Street, Suite B
Alexandria, VA 22314
http://www.migraines.org

National Headache Foundation
820 N. Orleans Street, Suite 217
Chicago, IL 60610
Tel: (888) NHF-5552
http://www.headaches.org

World Headache Alliance
41 Welbeck Street
WIG 8EA London, UK
http://www.w-h-a.org
email: mail@w-h-a.org

Acupuncture

American Academy of Medical Acupuncture
1970 E. Grand Avenue, Suite 330
El Segundo, CA 90245
Tel: (310) 364-0193
http://www.medicalacupuncture.org

**National Certification Commission for Acupuncture
and Oriental Medicine**
76 South Laura Street, Suite 1290
Jacksonville, FL 32202
Tel: (904) 598-1005
Fax: (904) 598-5001
http://www.nccaom.org

Biofeedback

Association for Applied Psychophysiology and Biofeedback
10200 W. 44th Avenue, Suite 304
Wheat Ridge, CO 80033
Tel: (800) 477-8892
http://www.aapb.org

Biofeedback Certification Institute of America
10200 West 44th Avenue, Suite 310
Wheat Ridge, CO 80033
Tel: (303) 420-2902
http://www.bcia.org

APPENDIX

233

Complementary & Alternative Medicine

The Mind/Body Medical Institute
Division of Behavioral Medicine
New England Deaconess Hospital
185 Pilgrim Road
Boston, MA 02215
Tel: (617) 732-9530

National Center for Complementary and Alternative Medicine/National Institutes of Health
Tel: (888) 644-6226
http://nccam.nih.gov

White House Commission on Complementary and Alternative Medicine Policy
Tel: (866) 512-1800
http://www.whccamp.hhs.gov

Guided Imagery

The Academy for Guided Imagery
10780 Santa Monica Boulevard, Suite 290
Los Angeles, CA 90025
Tel: (800) 726-2070
http://www.academyforguidedimagery.com

Hypnosis

The Society for Clinical and Experimental Hypnosis
http://www.sceh.us

The American Society of Clinical Hypnosis
140 N. Bloomingdale Road
Bloomingdale, IL 60108
Tel: (630) 980-4740
http://www.asch.net

**National Board for Certified Clinical
   Hypnotherapists, Inc.**
1110 Fidler Lane, Suite 1218
Silver Spring, MD 20910
Tel: (800) 449-8144
http://www.natboard.com

Massage Therapy

American Massage Therapy Association
500 Davis Street, Suite 900
Evanston, IL 60201-4695
Tel: (847) 864-0123
http://www.amtamassage.org

**National Certification Board for Therapeutic
   Massage and Bodywork**
1901 South Neyers Road, Suite 240
Oakbrook Terrace, IL 60181
Tel: (630) 627-8000
http://www.ncbtmb.com

The Rolf Institute
5055 Chaparral Court, Suite 103
Boulder, CO 80301
Tel: (800) 530-8875
http://www.rolf.org

Meditation

See also the **Recommended Reading** section on the following page.

**The Center for Mindfulness in Medicine, Health Care,
   and Society**
http://www.umassmed.edu/cfm/mbsr/

Mental Health

The American Psychological Association
750 First Street, NE
Washington, DC 20002-4242
Tel: (800) 474-2721
http://www.apa.org

National Institute of Mental Health (NIMH)
Science Writing, Press, and Dissemination Branch
6001 Executive Boulevard, Room 8184, MSC 9663
Bethesda, MD 20892-9663
Tel: (301) 443-4279
http://www.nimh.nih.gov

The National Mental Health Association
2000 N. Beauregard Street, 6th Floor
Alexandria, VA 22311
Tel: (800) 969-6642
Fax: (703) 684-5968
http://www.nmha.org

Sleep

National Sleep Foundation
1522 K Street NW, Suite 500
Washington, DC 20005
Tel: (202) 347-3471
http://www.sleepfoundation.org

Recommended Reading

The Relaxation Response, by Benson and Klipper. New York:
   Avon; 1976.

Beyond the Relaxation Response, by Benson and Proctor.
   New York: New York Times Books; 1984.

Healing Yourself: A Step-by-Step Program for Better Health Through Imagery, by Rossman. New York: Walker; 1987.

Healing With The Mind's Eye, by Samuels. New York: Random House; 1992.

Full Catastrophe Living: Using the Wisdom of Your Body and Mind to Face Stress, Pain, and Illness, by Kabat-Zinn. New York: Dell Publishing Group; 1990.

Minding the Body, Mending the Mind, by Borysenko. New York: Bantam Press; 1988.

Meditation as Medicine: Activate the Power of Your Natural Healing Force, by Khalsa. New York: Fireside Books; 2001

APPENDIX

Other Resources

Dr. Andrew Weil's Self Healing: Creating Natural Health for Your Body and Mind (website)

http://www.drweil.com

An excellent source on breathing techniques and background information on healing breathwork practices. Dr. Weil is also the author of numerous books on self-healing.

SAMPLE HEADACHE DIARY

Date	Time of headache	Duration of headache	Pain rating (0-10)	Other symptoms (i.e. nausea, fatigue)	Foods eaten prior to headache	Mood / stress prior to headache	Medications taken	Other interventions taken (i.e. rest, relaxation techniques)	Results of medication or interventions

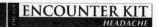

Patient Headache Diary

MIGRAINE IS TREATABLE

Migraine is treatable and sometimes preventable. Tracking headaches and headache "triggers" can assist in determining what helps and what brings on a migraine attack. Use this form to track your headaches and share the information with your doctor at your next visit.

USING THE PATIENT HEADACHE DIARY

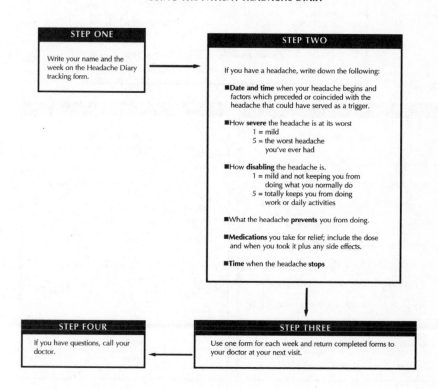

STEP ONE

Write your name and the week on the Headache Diary tracking form.

STEP TWO

If you have a headache, write down the following:

■**Date and time** when your headache begins and factors which preceded or coincided with the headache that could have served as a trigger.

■How **severe** the headache is at its worst
  1 = mild
  5 = the worst headache you've ever had

■How **disabling** the headache is.
  1 = mild and not keeping you from doing what you normally do
  5 = totally keeps you from doing work or daily activities

■What the headache **prevents** you from doing.

■**Medications** you take for relief; include the dose and when you took it plus any side effects.

■**Time** when the headache **stops**

STEP FOUR

If you have questions, call your doctor.

STEP THREE

Use one form for each week and return completed forms to your doctor at your next visit.

AMERICAN ACADEMY OF NEUROLOGY

Mnemonic Screening Tools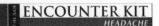

S-U-L-T-A-N-S

The mnemonic S-U-L-T-A-N-S can help with migraine diagnosis

1st Criteria
- **S**evere
- **U**ni**L**ateral
- **T**hrobbing
- **A**ctivity Worsens Headache

(need at least two from this list)

2nd Criteria
- **N**ausea
- **S**ensitivity to light/sound

(need one from this list)

Developed by Morris Maizels, MD, Kaiser Permanente

S-N-O-O-P-S

Headache Red Flags

- **S**ystemic Symptoms (fever, weight loss)

- **N**eurologic Symptoms or abnormal signs

  (confusion, impaired alertness or conciousness)

- **O**nset: sudden, abrupt or split second

- **O**lder: new onset or progressive headache,

  especially in patients >50 (giant cell arteritis)

- **P**revious headache history: first headache or

  new or different headache (change in attack

  frequency, severity or clinical features)

- **S**econdary Risk Factors (HIV, systemic cancer)

Developed by David Dodick, MD, Mayo Clinic Scottsdale

DEPRESSION

Two-question Screening for Depression

- During the past month, have you often been
  bothered by little interest or pleasure in doing
  things?
- During the past month, have you often been
  bothered by feeling down, depressed or
  hopeless?

S-A-L-S-A
4 vegetative signs of depression
- **S**leep disturbance
- **A**nhedonia
- **L**ow Self-Esteem
- **A**ppetite change

Migraine in a Minute

ENCOUNTER KIT
HEADACHE

MIGRAINE IN A MINUTE

Adapted from Morris Maizels, MD, Kaiser Permanente

Use the frequency of severe and mild headache and medication use to categorize patients as migraine (i.e.: episodic, severe), daily headache and/or medication overuse.

Q1. How often do you get severe headaches (i.e. without treatment it's difficult to function)?
This question alone identifies migraine. Any patient with severe headaches which are episodic should be assumed to have migraine.

Q2. How often do you get other (milder) headaches?
Daily headaches should always be evaluated for "worrisome" features. Patients with daily headaches (at times severe and migrainous) may have "transformed migraine," often due to medication overuse.

Q3. How often do you take headache relievers or pain pills?
Use of symptomatic medications more than 3 days/week represents medication overuse. The label, "drug rebound headache," should not be applied without a complete evaluation that has considered secondary and "worrisome" headaches. When drug rebound headache is recognized, symptomatic medications must be withdrawn for the patient to improve.

Q4. Has there been any recent change in your headaches?
The best screening question for "worrisome" headaches. A patient with a stable pattern of headache for 6 months has the same likelihood of an underlying tumor as a patient without headache.

Q5. How often do you miss work (or leisure activities) because of headache?
Good question for headache-related disability.

Q6. Are you satisfied with your current headache medicine?
Rapidly assesses acute therapy.

Q7. Are you on a preventive medicine for headache? If not, would you like to be?
Determines the patient's preference for prophylaxis.

AMERICAN ACADEMY OF NEUROLOGY

Glossary

A

Abortive medications: Medicines used to stop a migraine attack once it has started.

Acetaminophen: A mild analgesic used to abort migraine attacks. Can be purchased over the counter.

Acupressure: A Chinese traditional therapy using finger pressure at specific points along the body to treat stress and pain-related symptoms.

Acupuncture: A Chinese traditional therapy using fine needles inserted at specific points in the body to stimulate and regulate the flow of *chi* or vital energy to restore a healthy energy balance.

Amines: One of the building blocks of proteins. These substances have been implicated as triggers for migraines and are found in many foods that set off attacks.

Analgesic: Pain-relieving medication.

Antidepressant medications: These medications work to either enhance or alter chemicals in the brain. There are several different classes of these medications that vary depending on the mechanisms by which they work.

They work to improve mood as well as prevent pain. They are used in both psychiatry and neurology.

Antiepileptic medications: These medications work to prevent seizures, stabilize moods, and prevent pain. They are used in both psychiatry and neurology.

Arteriovenous malformation (AVM): An abnormal tangle of blood vessels, arteries, and veins in the brain. AVMs may bleed, cause seizures, focal neurological deficits, migraines, or no symptoms at all.

Autonomic nervous system: Includes the sympathetic and parasympathetic nervous systems that transmit nerve impulses from the central nervous system. This system controls blood pressure, pulse, and other automatic functions of the body.

B

Benign intracranial hypertension: A headache disorder characterized by increased pressure in the brain, often treated by removing cerebrospinal fluid. This disorder is usually accompanied by blurring of vision. Often patients are overweight and female.

Biofeedback: The use of electrical devices to recognize changes in body functions (heart rate, muscle tension) to achieve relaxation. Used to treat stress and pain-related conditions.

Blinded-placebo-controlled: When setting up clinical trials, researchers prefer to compare treatments using a blinded-placebo controlled trial. This involves assuring that neither the patient nor the researcher knows whether the patient is receiving the actual medication or a placebo (see **placebo**).

Blood pressure medication: Medicine used to control blood pressure as well as to prevent migraines.

Botulinum toxin (Botox®): A toxin produced by a bacterium that causes paralysis of muscles. This toxin may prevent migraines when injected into muscles of the face and neck.

Brain stem: A portion of the brain that is relatively primitive and controls the nerves that control facial expression, swallowing, hearing, eye movements, and sensation of the face and mouth. It is also the part of the brain that is believed to be implicated in the genesis of migraines.

Brain tumors: Tumors of the brain may be malignant or benign. The most common brain tumor is slow growing and benign and occurs more frequently in women. Many times these tumors cause no problems. Other, more aggressive tumors are much rarer.

Breathing techniques: Variety of techniques that use patterned breathing to achieve relaxation. Used to treat stress and pain-related conditions and achieve overall calm.

Bruxism: Grinding or clenching of the teeth, usually at night.

C

Calcitonin gene-related peptide: A neuropeptide that acts as a neurotransmitter to dilate blood vessels.

Carotid artery: One of the large vessels in the neck that provides blood to the brain.

Catecholamines: Brain chemicals that lower the pain threshold and result in the experience of more pain.

Central nervous system: The portion of the nervous system located in the spinal column and skull. It includes the brain and cranial nerves and spinal cord.

Cervical spine: The upper portion of the spine or neck. The spinal cord in this portion of the spine sends nerves to the arms and the back of the head.

Cervicogenic: Headaches that emanate from the irritation of nerves in the neck.

Channelopathy: An abnormality in the membranes of neurons, the cells in the brain, making them more excitable and susceptible to migraine triggers.

Chiropractic: The use of spinal manipulation to correct misalignments along the spine.

Chromosome 19p13: The chromosome implicated in familial hemiplegic migraine. This is a rare but interesting disorder of families whereby their migraines lead to paralysis. This disorder has allowed scientists to learn a great deal about the inheritance and pathophysiology of migraine.

Chronic migraine: A headache lasting 15 days or more per month for 3 months or more, and with no evidence of medication overuse.

Classical migraine: Another, older, name for **Migraine with aura**.

Claustrophobia: Fear or extreme discomfort in a dark and/or enclosed space.

Clinical hypnosis: Range of techniques to foster a state of awareness where relaxation and self-suggestions are achieved to bring about behavioral and emotional changes. Used commonly in pain, headaches, phobias, and anxiety.

Clinical psychologists: Specialists in the science of mind and behavior. They have a doctoral degree and provide various forms of psychotherapy and other clinical interventions to treat a wide variety of mental health and emotional disorders and concerns. Psychologists are not medical doctors and do not prescribe medication.

Clinical social workers: Professionals who provide a wide range of social and supportive services in hospitals and other health settings. Many clinical social workers or psychiatric social workers are also trained in providing psychotherapy or counseling services.

Clinical trial: A research study used to test a new medicine or treatment for a disease.

Cluster headache: A headache type that occurs primarily in men, which is characterized by severe pain lasting usually about 45 minutes, accompanied by nasal discharge and pain localized around or behind the eye. Headache episodes cluster temporally with episodes lasting several months with headache-free periods interspersed.

Common migraine: Another, older, name for **Migraine without aura**.

Comorbid: Diseases that occur together but are not related to each other.

Complementary and alternative medicine (CAM): A wide variety of healthcare practices and therapeutic approaches that fall outside the domain of conventional western medicine. CAM focuses on the diagnosis, prevention, and treatment of disease through the application of an assortment of practices such as biofeedback, acupuncture, massage, and chiropractic.

Complex partial seizures: Seizures that alter an individual's consciousness and may be associated with speech abnormalities and arm movements.

Cranial nerves: Nerves located in the head that control vision, facial expression, swallowing, hearing, eye movements, and sensation of the face and mouth. Most of these nerves emanate from the brain stem.

Creative visualization: The use of mental visual images to promote relaxation, healing, and changes in health and behavior.

D

Dangerous headache: A headache that is not typical for an individual and may be a harbinger of a potentially life-threatening process. All headaches thought to be dangerous should be evaluated or treated.

Diaphragmatic breathing: A breathing style that helps to fight stress. The breath originates from the diaphragm or belly instead of the chest.

Dipyridamole: A medicine that is used to keep your platelets from clotting together. This medicine is used to help prevent strokes.

E

Electroencephalography (EEG): A test performed by neurologists to assess brain waves. Performed by applying electrodes to the scalp to measure the electrical activity of the brain for 20 or more minutes. Patients may be asked to hyperventilate and/or have lights blinked rapidly in front of them to bring out abnormal brain waves. EEGs are used in the evaluation of seizures, alteration of consciousness, and coma.

Electrolytes: The substances in the blood that keep fluids in the body in balance. Extreme sweating, vomiting, and diarrhea may throw your electrolytes out of balance, making you feel weak and unable to function. Simple blood work will diagnose an imbalance, and IV fluids or even sport drinks may correct the abnormality.

Electromyographic (EMG) biofeedback: Technique that uses sensors attached to muscles that are tense during migraines to attain muscle relaxation.

Electromyography (EMG): A test performed by neurologists to assess muscle and nerve function. Fine needles are gently inserted into muscles to measure their electrical activity.

Empathize: The ability to relate to what another person feels or is going through.

Encephalitis: An infection of the brain matter.

Epidural hematoma: A traumatic blood clot of the brain that occurs soon after the traumatic incident and may be fatal if not treated. Usually causes rapid loss of consciousness, although headache may be experienced briefly as well.

Ergotamines: Medicines that are potent constrictors of blood vessels used to abort migraine attacks. These medicines can be inhaled nasally, injected, used as suppositories, or taken as pills.

F

Familial hemiplegic migraine: A rare inherited form of migraine characterized by weakness on one side of the body.

Fight-or-flight response: A state of arousal characterized by changes governed by the autonomic nervous system that include an increase in muscle tension, heart rate, blood pressure, and breathing.

Focal neurological deficit: Numbness, weakness, speech abnormalities, visual changes, difficulties walking, clumsiness, or any other problem with the body that can be attributed to the nervous system.

Fortification spectra: A visual phenomenon with a jagged appearance that usually begins prior to the onset of migraine pain. It usually begins centrally in the field of vision and gradually moves outward until it disappears.

Frontal and maxillary sinuses: Spaces in the bones of the face above the eyes (frontal) and below the eyes (maxillary) that may become congested and lead to infection and subsequent sinus headaches. These headaches are often confused with migraine headaches.

G

Gastric reflux: The regurgitation of stomach acids into the esophagus (the tube-like organ connecting the throat to the stomach). Medications and certain foods may cause this to occur.

Generalized seizures: Seizures during which patients lose consciousness, their limbs jerk, and they often urinate on themselves and bite their tongues.

Giant cell arteritis: An inflammation of the temporal artery that runs across the temple near the eye leading to pain, headache, and possible visual loss if not treated.

Guided imagery: The use of mental images, visualization, and imagination to promote healing or changes in health, emotions, and behaviors. Used for many stress and pain-related conditions.

Guillain-Barré Syndrome: A neurological disease where one becomes weak in a gradually ascending pattern. It may affect breathing as well. Neurologists take care of patients with this disease in the intensive care unit.

H

Headache danger signals: Symptoms and signs that may signal ominous etiologies of a headache. If you experience these types of symptoms, go to an emergency room or contact your physician.

Headache diary: A daily written record of events, foods, thoughts, and feelings that is used to identify a person's migraine triggers.

Hemicrania: Half of the brain or head. May also refer to one of the cerebral hemispheres.

Hemiparesis: Weakness on one side of the body; usually face, arm, and leg.

Herpes zoster: A rash or painful area of the face or trunk; also called shingles.

Homeopathic medicine: System of medicine based on concept of "like cures like"; symptoms are treated with minute doses of a substance that that would normally produce the same symptoms as the illness being treated.

Hypnosis: A range of techniques to foster a state of awareness where relaxation and self-suggestions are achieved to bring about behavioral and emotional changes.

I

Integrative medicine: The combination of complementary and alternative approaches and conventional medical treatment used to treat various medical, physical, and psychological disorders.

Intracranial lesions: Masses, tumors, abnormal blood vessels, blood clots, or other abnormalities located in the brain.

Intravenously: Administered by a catheter inserted into a vein.

L

Letdown migraine: Migraine episode that may occur after a period of emotional or physical stress and that frequently occurs on weekends. Also known as "weekend migraines."

Lorenzo's Oil: A movie about a rare neurological disease that afflicts children. This movie illustrates the role that neurologists play in caring for patients with rare and devastating neurological diseases.

Lou Gehrig's Disease (amyotrophic lateral sclerosis): The disease that struck down the baseball player Lou Gehrig. This disease causes a weakness in the muscles of the limbs and throat, rendering the patient unable to move, speak, and breathe on his or her own.

Lumbar puncture: A procedure done to obtain spinal fluid by inserting a needle into the base of the spine between vertebrae (also known as a spinal tap). The needle does not touch the spinal cord because it is below the level of the spinal cord, or nerves, but only extracts fluid. This fluid is then sent to a lab for analysis.

M

Massage therapy: Pressure, massage, and manipulation of muscle and tissue in the treatment of musculoskeletal pain.

Medication overuse headache: A headache that occurs when medications are used daily and then abruptly stopped.

Medi-speak: Tendency to speak using medical terms the listener may not understand.

Meditation: Process of focused attention to cultivate increased awareness.

Meninges: The tissues that envelope the brain matter. These tissues protect the brain, but may also become infected with viruses and bacteria leading to **meningitis**.

Meningioma: A relatively common benign brain tumor seen mostly in women.

Migraine without aura: A moderately severe to severe headache on one side of the head usually accompanied by sensitivity to noise and light, nausea and vomiting; it is throbbing in nature and lasts anywhere from four hours to seventy-two hours.

Migraine with aura: A migraine preceded by flashing lights, visual loss, or other visual or neurological phenomena. Also called classical migraine.

Mitochondria: Often called the "power houses" of a cell, these are the energy-producing structures in cells.

Monozygotic twin: Twins that share the same sex and genetic constitution; identical twins.

N

Naturopathic medicine: Health-care system that uses diet, herbs, and other natural methods to treat illness.

Neuralgia: Severe pain or tingling in the distribution of a nerve.

Neuromuscular massage: Technique that works by applying deep pressure to trigger points, a common cause of muscle pain in headache and myofascial disorders.

Neurons: The cells in the nervous system.

Neurotransmitters: The chemical messengers in the nervous system. These chemicals are involved in pain, emotion, mood, sensation, movement, and the special senses.

Nitric oxide: A molecule that is involved in dilating blood vessels.

Nitrite (nitrate): A potent vasodilator found in medications and many packaged and preserved foods, especially meats.

Nonsteroidal anti-inflammatory drug (NSAID): Medication used to abort migraines. Also used in many other pain syndromes where inflammation may be felt to play a role.

O

Optic nerve: The cranial nerve that conveys vision. The end of this nerve is actually visible to physicians when they look into an eye.

Osteopathy: School of medicine that provides comprehensive medical care. Osteopathic physicians prescribe medications and provide services the same as allopathic doctors, but pay special attention to joints, bones, muscles, and nerves.

P

Peripheral and central nervous system: The nervous system is composed of a central portion that includes the brain and spinal cord, and a peripheral portion that includes the peripheral nerves, nerve endings, and muscles.

Placebo: An inactive substance given, usually during a research trial, to compare its effect with the actual drug. Many have an effect from placebos due to suggestion, referred to as a placebo effect.

Placebo-controlled: A comparison of a drug or treatment against an inert substance (**placebo**).

Platelet aggregation: The tendency of the clotting cells (platelets) to get together and form clots. These clots may lead to strokes in the brain.

Polymyalgia rheumatica: A rheumatological disease characterized by weight loss, fever, muscle aches and pain, and on occasion, vision loss (temporal arteritis).

***Predator* effect:** A type of visual aura similar to the effect seen in the movie *The Predator* where an object appears to distort the background as though it is being viewed through ground glass.

Premenstrual syndrome (PMS): Bloating, moodiness, headache, cravings, and fatigue seen 1 to 3 days prior to the onset of menses.

Premonitory symptoms: Signs of an impending migraine.

Prevalence: The number of people who have a disease at any given point in time as a proportion of the total population.

Prophylactic medications: Medications used to prevent migraines and/or decrease the frequency and severity of your migraines. These medicines usually take several weeks to work and are usually used in combination with abortive migraine treatments.

Psychiatrist: A medical doctor who specializes in treating mental, emotional, and behavioral disorders such as depression and anxiety. Psychiatrists are physicians and thereby can prescribe medication to treat a wide variety of mental health problems.

Psychopharmacotherapy: The use of medication to treat psychiatric disorders, conditions, and symptoms.

Psychotherapy: A term used to describe a wide variety of talking and behavioral therapies to treat a variety of mental health and emotional conditions and disorders such as depression, anxiety, and adjustment concerns related to stress and relationships.

Q

Qi gong: Traditional Chinese approach using movements, breath-work, and meditation to maintain health.

R

Rebound headaches: Headaches that occur when a medication is taken daily to relieve pain and then withdrawn. The headache recurs with greater intensity due to the withdrawal of the medicine.

Reiki: Traditional Chinese form of touch-based energy healing.

Relaxation response: Physiological response associated with reduced stress and changes in heart rate, blood pressure, and breathing. The physiological and emotional opposite of the fight-or-flight response.

Relaxation techniques: A wide variety of techniques, including breath-work, meditation, guided imagery, and yoga, to promote relaxation and physical and mental well-being. Used commonly in the treatment of stress and pain-related conditions.

Riboflavin: Vitamin B_2. This vitamin has been found to be useful in decreasing the frequency and number of days of migraine attacks if taken regularly in doses of 400 mg.

Rolfing: A deep form of manipulation of the muscles and fascia that are often involved in musculoskeletal pain.

S

Scotoma: A dark spot in the field of vision in one eye. May be temporary or permanent.

Secondary headaches: Headaches due to a specific cause, such as tumor, stroke, or head trauma.

Seizure: Electrical discharges in the brain leading to alterations or loss of consciousness.

Selective serotonin reuptake inhibitors (SSRIs): A class of antidepressant medications that regulate the neurotransmitter serotonin in the brain.

Serotonin: A neurotransmitter involved in the regulation of moods and pain.

Serotonin or 5-hydroxytryptamine (5-HT) receptor: The receptor for serotonin that is very important in the migraine neurochemical pain cascade. Triptans work at this receptor to relieve pain.

Shiatsu: Form of acupressure to maintain good health and relaxation.

Sporadic hemiplegic migraines: Migraines that are accompanied by a weakness on one side or limb of the body.

Spreading cortical depression: A phenomena seen in brain cells when their activity becomes depressed immediately prior to the onset of the pain of a headache. This phenomenon is usually experienced by the migraineur as an aura or other visual or physical symptom prior to the onset of their headache.

Status migrainosis: A migraine that does not respond to your usual treatment and continues for a longer than usual time period. These migraines may last days to more than a week and require steroids or narcotics to break the pain.

Stepwise approach to migraine treatment: Method of treating migraines that entails starting with first-line, low-strength medicines, and increasing to stronger and more specific drugs until pain relief is achieved.

Stratified approach to migraine treatment: Method of treating migraines that entails starting with the most appropriate medication based on the patient's symptoms, lifestyle, and resources.

Stress: Caused by emotional, physical, and environmental changes, stress is the way our bodies and minds respond to the changes and demands upon us.

Stroke: Sudden or gradual onset of focal neurological deficits due to a blockage of blood vessels in the large vessels in the neck or brain or hemorrhage due to high blood pressure.

Subcutaneous injection: Injection of medication given directly below the skin.

Subdural hematoma: A traumatic blood clot of the brain that is often chronic and may lead to secondary headaches and seizures.

Swedish massage: Form of massage involving long strokes and kneading of muscle. Treats muscle tension and promotes overall relaxation.

Systemic diseases: Diseases that affect more than one organ system, such as high blood pressure, diabetes, and renal failure.

T

Tacrine: A medicine used to treat the symptoms of Alzheimer's disease.

Temporal arteritis: A rheumatological disease seen in older adults characterized by tender arteries in the temples and vision loss (partial or complete). May be associated with polymyalgia rheumatica.

Temporo-mandibular joint: The joint where the jaw meets the skull.

Tension headaches: Headaches that are bilateral, pressing, and of mild to moderate severity. Often occur in people who also have migraines.

The International Classification of Headache Disorders: A well-accepted classification used to diagnose headaches. This classification system is also used in research.

Traditional Chinese medicine: System of medicine dating back thousands of years. Integrates a variety of ancient and modern therapies including acupuncture, herbal medicine, and massage to treat a wide range of medical conditions.

Triage: The process of determining priority in treating patients.

Tricyclic antidepressants: A class of antidepressant medication also used to treat headache and other pain conditions.

Trigeminal neuralgia: The trigeminal nerve is the fifth cranial nerve; it controls sensation of the face. Abnormalities in this nerve may lead to a disorder characterized by severe pain and tingling in the distribution of this nerve.

Trigemino-vascular system: The system in the brain and brain stem that has been discovered to be the heart of the migraine generator. Neurochemical processes are believed to begin here and lead to the neurochemical cascade resulting in a migraine.

Trigger point: A spot in a muscle where if touched can elicit pain or radiation of pain. If injected with a steroid or anesthetic, this pain is relieved.

Triggers: Specific events or conditions that may trigger or provoke a migraine episode. May include certain foods, stress, weather conditions, or travel—among many other possibilities.

Triptan effect: Sensation of warmth, fullness in the throat, tingling in the arms and legs, dizziness, and nausea felt a short while after taking a triptan preparation.

Triptans: A revolutionary class of medications that act at the serotonin receptor to alleviate migraine pain.

U

Unilateral: Occurring on one side only.

Upper crossed syndrome: Upper body postural distortion believed to lead to cervicogenic and migraine headaches.

Urinary incontinence: Involuntary loss of urine due to a neurological cause (seizures, multiple sclerosis, spinal cord injury, etc.), urological causes, gynecological causes, coughing, laughing, etc.

V

Vascular: Having to do with blood vessels.

Vasoconstrictor: A medicine that causes blood vessels to constrict.

Vasodilation: Expansion of blood vessels.

Vesicles: Small blisters seen prior to the pain of shingles.

Viral meningitis: A viral infection of the tissues surrounding the brain.

W

Warfarin: A potent blood thinner used to prevent strokes and to prevent clots in heart patients. This medication also may put patients at risk for bleeding in the brain.

Weekend migraines: Also referred to as "letdown migraines," these are migraine episodes that occur typically following an intense build-up of stress.

Y

Yoga: A discipline that promotes physical, emotional, and spiritual well-being through posture, stretches, breathing, and meditative exercises.

Index

Italicized page locators indicate a figure; tables are noted with a *t*.

INDEX